Endorsements

Dr. Bob's natural health tips will take Christians to a higher level of optimal health.

—Jordan Rubin
New York Times best-selling author of *The Maker's Diet*
Founder, Garden of Life

As the senior pastor of two churches in two different major metropolitan cities, with more than 28,000 church members combined, it would be an understatement to say that I'm extremely busy! But I plan to live a long time to fulfill God's purpose for my life, so it's imperative that I maintain my health. If you want to live a longer and healthier life, *Dr. Bob's Guide to Optimal Health* makes it easier for you. This practical, user-friendly tool takes biblical principles and combines them with sound health and nutrition information to give you a daily plan designed to help you achieve optimal health. Let Dr. Bob show you how to transform your life. Your journey to a healthier you begins here!

—Dr. Creflo A. Dollar
Founder and Senior Pastor
World Changers Church International/
World Changers Church—New York

Dr. Bob's

GUIDE TO
OPTIMAL
HEALTH

Dr. Bob's

GUIDE TO

OPTIMAL
HEALTH

EXPANDED EDITION

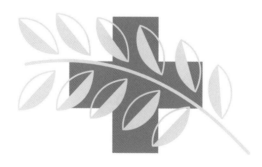

A God-Inspired, Biblically-Based 12 Month
Devotional to Natural Health Restoration

Dr. Robert DeMaria

The nutritional and health information in this book is based on the teachings of God's Holy Word, the Bible, as well as research and personal experiences by the authors and many others. The purpose of this book is to provide information and education about health. The authors and publisher do not offer medical advice or prescribe the use of diet as a form of treatment for sickness.

Because there is always some risk involved when changing diet and lifestyles, the author and publisher are not responsible for any adverse effects or consequences that might result. Please do not apply the teachings of this book if you are not willing to assume the risk. If you do use the information contained in this book without the approval of a health professional, you are prescribing for yourself, which is your constitutional right, but the author and publisher assume no responsibility.

DESTINY IMAGE. PUBLISHERS, INC.

P.O. Box 310, Shippensburg, PA 17257-0310

"Promoting Inspired Lives."

This book and all other Destiny Image, Revival Press, MercyPlace, Fresh Bread, Destiny Image Fiction, and Treasure House books are available at Christian bookstores and distributors worldwide.

For a U.S. bookstore nearest you, call 1-800-722-6774.

For more information on foreign distributors, call 717-532-3040.

Reach us on the Internet: www.destinyimage.com.

ISBN 13 TP: 978-0-7684-0328-2

ISBN 13 Ebook: 978-0-7684-8572-1

For Worldwide Distribution, Printed in the U.S.A.

9 10 11 / 22 21 20 19

The information provided in this book is with the understanding that the author is not liable for the misconception or misuse of information included. Every effort has been made to make this material as complete and accurate as possible. The author of this material shall have neither liability nor responsibility to any person or entity with respect to any loss, damage or injury caused or alleged to be caused directly or indirectly by the information contained in this manuscript. The information presented herein is not intended to be a substitute for medical counseling.

Some statistics and report information contained within are sourced through the Center for Science in the Public Interest (CSPI), a consumer advocacy organization that provides research and programs in health and nutrition.

Dedication

This book is dedicated to all the faithful in God's Kingdom who have been inspired to write. Like my good friend Myles Munroe says, "You all have a book inside of you; don't take it to the cemetery." Thanks to all of you who use the media to get God's message to the people. I pray this material will restore health in those who desperately need it.

Acknowledgments

In the Word of God, the Lord spoke a parable about building a structure and the work involved in measuring and evaluating the products necessary for a complete and solid structure. I would like to personally acknowledge and thank a few of the many who have helped make this project a success:

First, I acknowledge my wife and best friend in the whole world, Deb. She has been the wind beneath my wings for over thirty years and has unselfishly supported my entire life. I have been blessed with two of the finest sons anyone could ask for. Dominic and Anthony will be pillars in their generation. They have been a source of parental pride and pleasure and a real inspiration.

I could not have completed this project without the help of Kim Plaso, who typed the entire text from my handwritten notes. The editing expertise of Laura Meyer was very helpful.

I would like to acknowledge all those who reviewed the manuscript, especially Louis Kayatin, the first pastor to impact my life. Also Bob Harrison—he has been a blessing to the Christian and secular business community, connecting people.

Pastors Paul Endrei's, Ricardo Johnson's, and Jeffrey Paul's knowledge of the Word assisted me during the development process.

I want to thank all the patients who wrote personal testimonies in response to reaching their goals of optimal health.

I am extremely appreciative for the hundreds of thousands of patients I have had the opportunity to personally administer to since beginning my practice in 1978.

And thank you to each and every one of the prayer warriors who strengthen me.

The Value of a Friend

Two are better than one,
Because they have a good reward for their labor;
For if they fall, one will lift up his companion.
But woe to him who is alone when he falls,
For he has no one to help him up.
Again, if two lie down together, they will keep warm;
But how can one be warm alone?
Though one may be overpowered by another,
two can withstand him,
And a threefold cord is not quickly broken.
Ecclesiastes 4:9-12

Contents

Foreword

If the physical body is truly a temple, then its protection, maintenance, preservation, and care are the responsibility of the host. No one can love or will love your body more than you. Over the years, as a pastor and spiritual leader, I have magnified and focused on the soul and spiritual aspects of the human and in many ways downplayed and almost ignored the role, value, importance, and significance of the physical body. However, after more than thirty years of research, study, and personal development, I have concluded that the Creator's purpose and role for the physical body places it as the most important component in the human earthly journey.

When the apostle Paul says that we should offer our bodies as living sacrifices (see Rom. 12:1), he is telling us to bring our bodies under management—to get them under control. Stop drinking or stealing or smoking or lying or doing drugs. Stop engaging in illicit and immoral sexual activity. Stop playing around with pornography. Break off unhealthy relationships. Bring our bodies under subjection. Keep our bodies and minds pure.

It is important that we learn to manage our bodies and get them in order because they are our legal houses. If we lose them, we cannot do anything else. We can't serve God effectively if we are addicted to tobacco or alcohol. We can't fulfill our potential if, by age thirty, we are sick and have cancer in our lungs. The Lord cannot bless us if we are shacking up with someone or abusing our minds or bodies in any way or living in any manner that is contrary to His revealed will. He wants us to bring our bodies under subjection and present them to Him as *living* sacrifices from which He can receive great glory and honor.

The command by God to keep our bodies pure is motivated by His need for our bodies in order to accomplish His will on earth. He designed our bodies for Himself, and He needs them as legal agencies for heavenly involvement on the planet. Here is a verse you may not have read in Paul's writings: *"The body is not meant for sexual immorality, but for the Lord, and the Lord for the body"* (1 Cor. 6:13 NIV).

Paul says next in Romans 12 that we need to *"be transformed by the renewing of* [our] *mind*[s]." What does he mean? His point is that even though, as believers, we have been born again, we still have a mental problem. We have the Holy Spirit, but not the *spirit* of the Holy Spirit. We have the anointing, but not the *spirit* of the anointing. We need to change our thinking. The Greek word *metamorphoo* (from which comes the English word *metamorphosis*) literally means to make a complete and total change. The transformation that Paul talks about here involves a complete revolution of our mental state.

In this book, Robert DeMaria provides a sound, practical, principle-centered approach to recovering, maintaining, protecting, and preserving our bodies with the intent of living out our days, fulfilling our earthly assignments, and glorifying God in our bodies. I was gripped by the profound yet simple wealth of information presented in a people-friendly way that does not complicate issues with language beyond the layman. Robert leaps over complex technical terms and conveys the simple precepts that lead the reader to the well of the good, healthy lifestyle.

I recommend this book, and I challenge you to read it with an open heart and discover the biblical path to health and wellness.

—Dr. Myles E. Munroe
Founder, President, and Senior Pastor of Bahamas Faith Ministry
Author, *Understanding Your Potential* and *Discovering the Kingdom*

Preface

The following pages have been inspired by the Holy Spirit. I have always enjoyed reading a daily devotional from a variety of sources in the Christian community. Some of my favorites are historical greats, including Smith Wigglesworth and Oswald Chambers. Reading their spiritual insights has been inspiring for my own walk with the Lord. The Holy Spirit—who filled them so mightily—overflows through their words, keeping their insights alive today.

I was reading one of my favorite modern-day writers—I have many—when the Holy Spirit stopped me and told me to write this book. Each tip for optimal health has been inspired from above. I prayed over every one of the daily nuggets and natural prescriptions as I was writing them, knowing that lives would be impacted today and into the future. Your health is serious and important. Satan wants you to be sick—to keep you from receiving and becoming all that God intends for you. Jesus came to set you *free*—free from bondage and illness.

We are the temple of the Holy Spirit. Jesus is coming back for an awesome Bride. You will be ready.

Helpful Tips for Using
the Daily Guide & Devotional

The Lord has directed my steps while writing this book for you. He has provided the opportunities that produced the life-changing tips that I am sharing with you—compiled over my thirty years of experience in the healthcare field.

Jesus had twelve disciples in His main group of followers. His inner circle—James, Peter, and John—were part of His very close group of friends. My suggestion to you is to prayerfully seek two others who will participate with you over the next twelve months to reach your goal of optimal health. Proverbs 27:17 says, *"As iron sharpens iron, so a man sharpens the countenance of his friend."* Creating accountability and support will enhance your experience.

This devotional guide contains specific health-enhancing sections consisting of twenty-one-day patterns. Each day provides Bible verses and health tips that add quality to your life. For example, the first pattern focuses on the importance of adding or increasing water in your daily routine. Common-sense tips and proven medical results about water are provided.

Each day you can journal your feelings, read about specific problem areas, and learn a natural prescription health tip. Other patterns include mealtimes, children's health, and the topics listed on the Contents page. A "natural prescription for health" is included daily. An example: Eating in the morning is similar to fueling the fire in your furnace.

I also provide comments and concepts for your self-assessment. This is not win-or-lose assessment—it is a proactive approach to add to your daily routine. Each pattern, as it is added to your daily routine, will create a new you, and you will soon be saying, "I feel great!"

My website provides additional information and resources for you to use on your journey to optimal health. There is also a message board available where you can post your positive experiences and helpful hints for others.

This is an interactive guide. Meditate on what the Holy Spirit is speaking to you each day. Read God's Word daily.

For the best results, do not jump ahead in the book. After you've completed the twelve-month guide, you can review and study areas of particular interest.

Start by completing the initial Natural Health Assessment questionnaire. This will be your foundation on which to measure your progress after six and twelve months. Weigh yourself. Have someone take your blood pressure. It is even a good idea to have a fasting chemistry profile completed now. You need to monitor your body signals (pain, bowel movements, and so forth). Remember, this is going to be a positive experience.

The guide focuses on whole, organic foods. Do not feel obligated to adjust your budget. I have seen families with poor health and obesity patterns minimize their restaurant meals and achieve positive results. It is obvious looking around on any evening in your community; the American public enjoys eating their meals outside of the home. Consumers spend more than forty-six percent of their food dollars on freshly prepared food away from home.[1] Shift to family-produced wholesome meals. With some pre-planning, you and your family can achieve optimal health.

Do not self-diagnose or treat yourself with the suggestions made in this book. Although thousands have proven the advice true, seek the opinion of your healthcare provider before making any dramatic changes. I have treated thousands over my career using the information I am presenting to you. Regardless of my experience, it is always prudent on your part to talk to the healthcare provider of your choice in whom you have confidence—one who has a reputation of helping patients naturally.

The Bible is filled with key words and statements that promote life. I have included short, documented studies to validate my research. My patients gladly participated by adding their testimonies. You will thoroughly enjoy this life-changing experience. Tell a friend—be blessed!

—"Dr. Bob"
America's Drugless Care Doctor
www.druglessdoctor.com

Natural Health Assessment Questionnaire

This Natural Health Assessment has been designed to create optimal health. Take time to assess your current state of health. Then take the assessment again after six months to track your progress.

Health Assessment

How many of these health problems/symptoms do you have? (Check as many as apply.)

_____ Difficulty getting up in the morning

_____ Continual fatigue, not relieved by sleep and rest

_____ Lethargy, lack energy to perform normal, daily activities

_____ Sugar cravings

_____ Salt cravings

_____ Allergies

_____ Digestion problems

_____ Increased effort needed for everyday tasks

_____ Decreased interest in sex

_____ Decreased ability to handle stress

_____ Increased time needed to recover from illness, injury, or traumas

_____ Light-headed or dizzy feeling when standing up quickly

_____ Low emotional mood

_____ Less enjoyment or happiness with life

_____ Increased Premenstrual Syndrome symptoms

_____ Symptoms worsen if meals are skipped or inadequate

_____ Thoughts are less focused, brain fog

_____ Memory is poor

_____ Decreased tolerance for stress, noise, disorder

_____ Not fully awake until after 10 a.m.

_____ Afternoon low between 3 and 4 p.m.

_____ Feel better after supper

_____ Get a "second wind" in the evening and stay up late

_____ Decreased ability to get things done—less productive

_____ Have to keep moving—"If I stop, I get tired"

_____ Feeling overwhelmed by all that needs to be done

_____ It takes all my energy to do what I have to do—there's none left over for anything or anyone else.

_____ Date

_____ Date

_____ Date

Refreshing Water

Water promotes life. In the activity of daily living, many do not drink adequate amounts of pure water. Water bathes the cells and helps eliminate toxins. Start each day with a measured amount of water in a container and drink from it throughout the day. One formula to calculate how much water to drink is to take your body weight and divide that number by four. That number is the minimal number of ounces you should consume.

Do this for life…and for the rest of your life.

Day 1

Water Refreshes the Body

And the Spirit of God was hovering over the face of the waters (Genesis 1:2).

Water is essential for life. God refers to water in one of the very first Bible verses. The human body requires water to function at the cellular level. Water is necessary for proper digestion and elimination. Hunger pains may be a cry for water instead of food. Water is also found in fruits and vegetables.

Consuming soda, tea, and coffee actually creates a toxic fluid state in the body. Water is nature's way of cleaning the system. Water from a pure source (preferably reverse osmosis) is the best—daily drinking a minimum of one quart of water per 150 pounds of body weight.

Natural Prescription for Health: Start your day with a cup of hot water and lemon. This is an excellent liver cleansing stimulant.

Personal Thoughts/Goals:

_____

_____

_____

_____

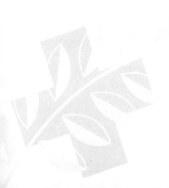

Day 2

Happy Heart, Clear Skin

...And while [Uzziah] *was angry with the priests, leprosy* [skin eruptions]
broke out on his forehead (2 Chronicles 26:19).

Skin not only protects us from the elements and helps maintain body temperature with active surface area for evaporation, but is it also an important part of detoxification. Your body is constantly looking for ways to eliminate by-products of metabolism and toxic waste buildup.

Patients with chronic skin eruptions, from acne to psoriasis, commonly have one or two major primary causes. Toxic backup from lack of pure water consumption is by far the leading cause of skin eruptions. Clean machines always work better. An overloaded, toxic liver is the second leading reason there are issues with skin. Emotional stresses, including anger, can put additional pressure on the liver to deal with the emotional response and chemical overload. Also, dairy consumption may be precipitating your teen's acne.

Increase water intake and eat raw carrots. Carrots are an excellent source of vitamin A that can be used by the skin and liver to promote a clean machine.

Natural Prescription for Health: Adequate water consumption is necessary for healthy skin no matter what the age. Do not count soda or coffee as water.

Personal Thoughts/Goals:

_____

_____

_____

_____

Day 3

The Walk by the Sea

Again, departing from the region of Tyre and Sidon, He came through the midst of the region of the Decapolis to the Sea of Galilee (Mark 7:31).

Jesus walked around and over the Sea of Galilee. My memory of being in the center of the sea still creates goose bumps. You can see the same hills and geography Jesus saw two thousand years ago. Even walking by a saltwater sea or any fresh body of water (the Sea of Galilee is fresh water) is beneficial for body cleansing.

Ocean waves create a negative ion charge. This promotes health and healing. The negative ions pull unwanted toxins from the body via the lymphatic system and literally charge you up. Your body absorbs minerals from the ocean. Aging, from my observation, creates a need for easily assimilated minerals. Hot mineral springs and even a home mineral bath is beneficial, since minerals can be absorbed through the skin.

Natural Prescription for Health: Swimming in bromine/chlorine-treated pools and hot tubs tends to deplete iodine. For a natural source of iodine, choose sea vegetables from an organic source. Shower de-chlorinators are an excellent option to reduce shower sourced chlorine

Personal Thoughts/Goals:

_____

_____

_____

_____

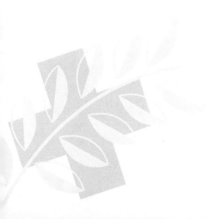

Day 4

What Do I Eat and Drink?

*Look at the birds of the air, for they neither sow nor reap nor gather into barns; yet your heavenly Father **feeds** them. Are you not of more value than they?*
(Matthew 6:26, emphasis added).

God's Word says, "Do not worry about what you should eat or drink" (see Matt. 6:31). Do you worry a lot? Give all your yokes to the Lord. Worry, crying without reason, sore muscles, and depression may be a sign that you need to eat more whole grains with complex B's versus white, synthetic, enriched foods.

I recommend you eat food that is God-made, not human-made. Keep it pure and simple. Eat foods that decay and spoil—food that needs to be consumed in a few days. Avoid processed foods. Start your day off by replacing pastries and gluten cereals with one half of a red apple with two teaspoons of organic almond butter, a poached egg, or quinoa. Gluten-based grains—including rye, wheat, oats, and barley—may be creating health challenges. Drink herbal teas, hot water with lemon, and caffeine in the morning only. Have a midmorning veggie snack such as celery, carrots, cherry tomatoes, cucumbers, or raw nuts. For lunch, try mixed greens with protein along with olive or flax oil and select herbs that you like. Vegetables, raw or steamed, along with a protein of your choice are great for dinner. No fruit after a meal. Any fruit, canned or fresh, will sit on top of the digesting protein and complex carbohydrates that are being digested first. They will sit there and putrefy like compost, causing indigestion. Homemade sweet items on a Sunday afternoon can be a real treat. Eat sweets *alone*—not in combination with other food. See pages 119–120, Food Combinations.

Be blessed! Ask the Lord to enlarge your capacity to create and enjoy the full spectrum of foods He created for us to enjoy.

Natural Prescription for Health: Eat one fresh organic vegetable, raw or steamed, that you have not tried before.

Personal Thoughts/Goals:

_____

_____

Day 5

So Many Choices

*A righteous man who falters before the wicked is like a murky spring
and a polluted well* (Proverbs 25:26).

Choosing a quality water source may not have been significant to you years ago; however, it is very important today. I recently listened to a couple who have digestive distress tell me how their municipal water (from their faucet) appears to affect their health. Their community water department issued a statement in their local newspaper about high "normal" substances in a mandatory report.

The water supply in my local municipality has contaminants at the extreme high end of "normal." Another local community has a higher-than-normal number of multiple sclerosis cases—possibly linked to a toxic source entering the water supply. I also have patients with well water who develop depression and emotional dysfunction. Be aware of your source of drinking and cooking water.

I encourage my patients to drink "reverse osmosis" filtered water. Spring water may have high levels of contaminants. Always check the purity of your water.

Natural Prescription for Health: Do not drink water that tastes, smells, or looks particulate. Tap water that has an odor of chlorine in the winter months should be avoided.

Personal Thoughts/Goals:

_____

_____

_____

_____

Day 6

Drink Only Water

*Wine makes you mean, beer makes you quarrelsome—a staggering drunk
is not much fun* (Proverbs 20:1 MSG).

It is a known fact that water is essential for a quality life. Motivating individuals to drink even a minimum amount can be challenging.

Alcohol, on the other hand, creates physical and emotional issues regardless of spiritual conviction and is commonly consumed in social and private settings. I am aware of research reports released that promote the efficacy of moderate alcohol consumption. The word *moderation* with alcohol, though, is like telling a child to have only one piece of candy.

Does alcohol interfere with your relationship with Jesus? When I, through the power of the Holy Spirit, was released from alcohol's grip on my life, the Holy Spirit replaced the alcohol desire with His presence and wisdom. I pray that my personal experience of overcoming will encourage the one who needs to be released.

Natural Prescription for Health: Alcohol consumption creates additional stress on an already overworked liver. The liver is your recycle organ; keep it pure.

Personal Thoughts/Goals:

_____

_____

_____

_____

Day 7

Stop Kidney Stones

Most people who suffer with kidney stones made of calcium oxalate (the most common kind) excrete too much calcium in their urine. So for years, doctors have told them to cut back on calcium. Now a new study has shown that advice was wrong. Eating less animal protein and using less salt works far better.[2]

Over five years, forty men who ate 50 grams of animal protein and 2,500 milligrams to 3,000 milligrams of sodium a day were half as likely to get another kidney stone as twenty-eight men who were told to eat no more than 400 milligrams of calcium.

The lower-protein, lower-salt diet reduced both calcium and oxalate in the men's urine. In contrast, the lower-calcium diet reduced calcium, but *increased* oxalate (probably because there was too little calcium to bind the oxalate in the intestine).

Natural Prescription for Health: If you've had a kidney stone made of calcium oxalate and you excrete excess calcium, limit your protein from meat, seafood, poultry, milk, cheese, and other dairy products to about 50 grams a day. The US Recommended Daily Allowance for protein is 50 grams, and that includes protein from breads, cereals, beans, and other plant foods. So the 50 gram limit on animal protein isn't exactly a low-protein diet.

And keep your sodium as close as possible to 2,400 milligrams a day (that's half what many Americans eat).

> Before I began care with Dr. DeMaria, I had gone to the hospital with chest pains. My liver enzymes were very high, and the doctor was talking about removing my gallbladder. Dr. Bob suggested that I start taking cleansing supplementation to clean up my liver that was toxic. I also started eating beets. After receiving care for about one month, I had my blood work done again. My liver enzymes were back to normal. My chest pains as well as my stomach pains were gone. Also, the brown spots on my face disappeared. —Mary Lou Bors

Personal Thoughts/Goals:

_____

_____

_____

Day 8

A Cup of Cold Water

And whoever gives one of these little ones only a cup of cold water in the name of a disciple, assuredly I say to you, he shall be no means lose his reward (Matthew 10:42).

Water purifies the body. Jesus was quite aware that water provides life and is required for all ages. I encourage my patients to drink a minimum of one quart of water from a clean source daily. Your body size determines the volume you need. It has been suggested to drink one-half ounce of water for every pound of weight.

Children who drink commercially-made juice, which is often sweetened with high fructose corn syrup, may develop health issues. Please become more aware of what your family and friends offer your children as a beverage. Carbonated beverages and soft drinks are devastating. One twelve-ounce can of soda contains nearly ten teaspoons of sugar. The immune system is paralyzed for hours after eating or drinking sugar. Water purifies the body. It is also a more satisfying thirst quencher.

Natural Prescription for Health: In addition to purified water, there are several healthier options from which to choose. Select grape juice sweetened spritzers as a soda option and herbal tea with fresh mint leaves in place of coffee.

Personal Thoughts/Goals:

_____

_____

_____

_____

Day 9

What Is Your Water Source?

*Now **Jacob's well** was there. Jesus therefore, being wearied from His journey, sat thus by the well...* (John 4:6, emphasis added).

Well water was a source of life and an oasis in the old covenant. Water is life. Patches of green in Israel's wilderness are localized around wells. The ground water several thousand years ago did not have high concentrations of herbicides, pesticides, and fertilizers, as is the case today. Do you drink well water? Did you ever drink well water as a child or at school?

I have patients who bathe in well water, but do not drink it, thinking that it is only harmful if they drink it. Results of their hair tissue mineral analysis reveal that even bathing in well water caused them to have toxic lead and iron levels. Depression and other emotional and physical conditions including liver, kidney, and skin reactions can result because of well water consumption. I would suggest a quality water purifier if you use water from ground tables and cisterns.

Natural Prescription for Health: Water sources should be tested, including treated municipal sources, for toxic material if you have challenging health conditions.

Personal Thoughts/Goals:

_____

_____

_____

_____

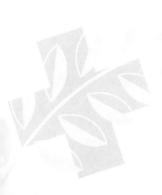

Day 10

Protect Yourself From Worldwide Pollution

Because the creation itself also will be delivered from the bondage of corruption into the glorious liberty of the children of God. For we know that the whole creation groans and labors with birth pangs together until now (Romans 8:21-22).

Creation groans, anxiously awaiting the return of Jesus. We live in a global community. Pollution from around the world settles in distant landing spots. Your liver is the critical organ to process the various pollutants. You need to be conscious of this and be disciplined to minimize the direct toxins you put into your body. Soda, prescription medication, processed food, or any human-made composition may stress your filter system.

Water filtration plants are not designed to clear modern petrochemical-based prescription medication. Mutated fish are a part of the ecosystem in areas where the water is sourced from ground water. Focus on drinking your daily water intake from a pure source. I do not promote distilled water. I have seen from practice experience that patients who drink distilled water appear to have challenges when testing muscle strength.

Natural Prescription for Health: Eliminate artificially sweetened beverages from your home and your daily diet.

Personal Thoughts/Goals:

_____

_____

_____

_____

Day 11

A Blessed Memory

Blessings are on the head of the righteous.... The memory of the righteous is blessed...
(Proverbs 10:6-7).

Through faith in Christ, God's righteousness is imputed or granted to believers (see Titus 3:5). Christians are encouraged to pursue the interests of God's righteous Kingdom. Regardless of your socioeconomic position, sex, race, or culture, a modern epidemic is loss of memory. Where did I put my keys? Did you see my glasses? I can't find my pen. A sign of memory loss—or poor focus?

The brain center for memory is called the Hippocampus. It is a major storage center for zinc. Zinc is depleted by wheat, soy, and sugar. Aluminum, which has been the subject of memory loss research, has an affinity for soy! My experience with hair analysis is that aluminum is elevated with stressed adrenal glands. Liver congestion from processed food consumption affects mental quickness. Female patients have memory resets during hormone fluctuations. Sugar consumption short-circuits the brain.

Natural Prescription for Health: Limit soy consumption and read labels. Add zinc-rich raw pumpkin seeds to your raw nut salad.

Personal Thoughts/Goals:

_____

_____

_____

_____

Day 12

Dead Sea Clay

And Lot lifted his eyes and saw all the plain of Jordan, that it was well watered everywhere...like the garden of the Lord... (Genesis 13:10).

Sodom and Gomorrah were flourishing cities at the time of their destruction, but they had detached themselves from the fear of God. The remains of their sin and demise have resulted in a present-day flourishing tourist attraction. The Dead Sea experience is quite mind-stretching. The water's mineral salt content is so high that you cannot become submerged without great effort. For an additional fee, you are provided with clay so you can literally take a "purifying" mud bath. What humanity had devised for evil, God used for good. The mineral salt in the black clay is quite a sight when applied on the skin. The physiology of the clay draws toxins and impurities out of the skin. Applying the mud as a mask on the face improves complexion, and a periodic mud bath goes a long way to restoring health. The Dead Sea is now an oasis in the desert, where people can benefit from the natural properties of salt and mud.

Natural Prescription for Health: Soak your feet in hot Epsom salt water and enjoy the natural release of toxic cellular debris. Do this weekly if you have swollen joints.

Personal Thoughts/Goals:

_____

_____

_____

_____

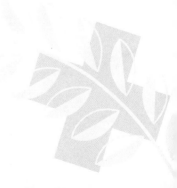

Day 13

Fluid Retention—Dropsy (Kidney Failure)

And behold there was a certain man before Him who had dropsy....
And He...healed him, and let him go (Luke 14:2,4).

Little healing was done in Nazareth because of little faith. Jesus healed all who had the faith to be healed. Dropsy, not a common term today, can be caused by a variety of reasons. *Fluid accumulation, swelling, edema,* and *swollen ankles* are more common terms used today. Diuretics are commonly prescribed to treat the *symptoms* of excessive fluid. This may surprise you, but increasing water from a pure source can release water accumulation in tissues by eliminating toxins accumulated from poor food choices. Heart and kidney function should be evaluated by a skilled, experienced healthcare provider if chronic, long-lasting swelling exists.

Increasing protein consumption often relieves the body of extra fluid. Fresh parsley is an excellent kidney purifying herb. Try adding it to your salads or make parsley tea with hot water. We support heart function with low dosage, cold-processed nutritional supplements and see reduced swelling as a result. I check all patients for proper alignment of the spinal segments associated with heart and kidney function. Correction aids restoration.

Natural Prescription for Health: Fresh parsley in your salad promotes kidney function. White potatoes which are considered a nightshade may create water retention or dropsy; yams and sweet potatoes would be a better choice.

Personal Thoughts/Goals:

_____

_____

_____

_____

Day 14

Carbonated Beverages and Soft Drinks Increase Body Weight

Drinking more soda these days? Watch out.

Researchers tracked more than fifty thousand women for four years. Those who went from drinking no more than one soft drink a week to at least one a day gained roughly ten pounds over the four-year period. A jump in fruit drink intake was also linked to weight gain, but diet soft drinks were not.

In a separate analysis of ninety thousand, those who drank soda or fruit drinks at least once a day had nearly twice the risk of diabetes compared to people who drank those beverages less than once a month. Though the soda drinkers also weighed more and ate more, that didn't entirely explain their higher risk.

Natural Prescription for Health: This study[3] can't prove that soda (or fruit drinks) cause more weight gain or diabetes than other foods. But it's one more reason to think twice before you reach for another 250-calorie bottle of soda; drink water instead.

> When I first came to see Dr. DeMaria, I had headaches, severe seasonal allergies, and high blood pressure. I took a lot of different headache medications and over-the-counter and prescription allergy medications. It was hard to break a lifetime of bad eating choices, but I have tried, and I've also learned that I was taking too many of the wrong kind of pills for my health problems. The diet changes and natural supplements do more, much more, than what my other doctor was doing for my problems. We all owe it to ourselves to try a natural lifestyle. —Janis Martin

Personal Thoughts/Goals:

_____

_____

_____

_____

Day 15

Drink Living Water

And the Spirit and the bride say, "Come!" And let him who hears say, "Come!"
And let him who thirsts come. Whoever desires, let him take the water of life freely
(Revelation 22:17).

The desire for water is an inborn need required for survival. Cells in the body are bathed in water. Jesus spoke about thirsting for Him as living water.

Persistent unhealthy body signals such as constipation, headaches, skin rashes, bad breath, sinusitis, and so forth, may all be alarms that your body needs more pure water. Here is a jolt. Water is not tea, soda, coffee, juice, milk, alcohol, or sport drinks. Water is pure and clear with nothing added. I encourage my patients to start the day off with a measured amount of water in a quart container; room temperature is preferred. As mentioned previously, a simple rule that can be modified for your need is to consume at least one-half ounce of water per pound of body weight. Do not exceed one hundred ounces in a day.

Natural Prescription for Health: Drink water one-half hour before or after meals because water may dilute stomach fluids needed for digestion. *Limited* sips (up to 4 ounces) during meal time will not interfere with digestion.

Personal Thoughts/Goals:

_____

_____

_____

_____

Day 16

Pay for Water?

We pay for the water we drink... (Lamentations 5:4).

Water is mentioned in God's Word in the beginning. Water is a purifier. Water is found in nearly every cell of the body. It is necessary for functions that we normally are not aware of until there is a breakdown. Most people mistake the craving for water as hunger and eat food when they should actually be drinking more water. Try it the next time you think you are hungry—drink eight ounces of pure water instead.

I never would have thought growing up that I would actually purchase water to drink. Water was only a turn of the knob away. Now, toxic wastes, poor filtration, and chemical neutralizers have all but made fresh water a precious commodity. In fact, there are locations in the US where fresh water supplies are legally contested. Water purchased in retail outlets costs more than gasoline—a gallon of pure water may cost nearly thirty dollars.

Do not miss an opportunity to drink water daily. It will improve chronic sinusitis and constipation.

Natural Prescription for Health: Drink water that is room temperature. Drink pure water before or after meals. Do not drink tap water that has not been purified.

Personal Thoughts/Goals:

_____

_____

_____

_____

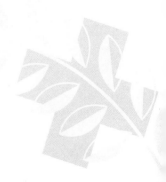

Day 17

The Lord Uses Ordinary People for Extraordinary Assignments

And Jethro, the priest of Midian, Moses' father-in-law, heard of all that God had done for Moses and for Israel, His people (Exodus 18:1).

God's Word is full of amazing, supernatural events. God can use the simple and the strong. I've noticed that extraordinary responsibility and opportunity for achievement were given to individuals with ordinary life experiences. Moses was under Pharaoh's covering for forty years, Joseph spent years managing a prison, and Paul was a Pharisee of Pharisees.

Are you ready for the next level? Replicate what you have gleaned and learned up to this point through your inner and extended circle of influence. Do not be judgmental. In a loving manner suggest more water. This is the single most important advice you can give. Answer comments such as, "I don't like the taste of water" with "Here, enjoy this water from a purified source. It will bless you with good health." An additional blessing would be to add an organic lemon to the refreshing glass of water. Your new assignment is going to *stretch you* into an environment where people want everything done for them. Now is the time to share your healthy thinking!

Natural Prescription for Health: Share with one person what you have learned about how important water is for a healthy body. Drink more water from a reliable, pure source.

Personal Thoughts/Goals:

_____

_____

_____

_____

Day 18

White Lamb's Wool Teeth

Your teeth are like a flock of sheep which have come up from the washing...
(Song of Solomon 6:6).

The lamb is used as a visual metaphor to explain the Kingdom of God. White represents purity, cleanliness, a state of complete wholeness. White teeth are a sign of optimal body function. Yellow tinted teeth usually appear with sluggish thyroid function. The thyroid gland has many functions, one being to keep calcium moving. Are your teeth yellow? Having them whitened professionally or with an over-the-counter product may not be a healthy decision—it is similar to short-circuiting the oil alert red light on your car's instrument panel.

Do you have cold hands or feet? Is your hair thin, sparse, and coarse? You may have low thyroid function. Take your basal armpit temperature first thing in the morning before you get out of bed or move around. Your temperature should be 97.8 degrees or above. If it is lower, I would suggest taking the following supplements: organic kelp (6 to 9 daily); calcium (6 daily); organic iodine (1 or 2 daily); flax (1 tablespoon per 100 pounds of body weight). Cell therapy with thyroid tissue will assist thyroid restoration. Continue the protocol until your temperature elevates and your thyroid functions properly.

Natural Prescription for Health: Take your basal armpit temperature for three mornings in a row. This simple procedure is a monitor for optimal body function.

Personal Thoughts/Goals:

_____

_____

_____

_____

Day 19

Satisfying Thirst

O God, You are my God; early I will seek you. My soul thirsts for You. My flesh longs for You in a dry and thirsty land where there is no water (Psalm 63:1).

God wants a relationship with us so intently that He relates it to the desire to satisfy thirst. Have you ever been so thirsty that your tongue feels like it is sticking to the roof of your mouth? Water is necessary for life. Without water from a pure source, we will die.

Water is not coffee, tea, fruit juice, chocolate milk, or any commercial product with a long list of additives. Sport drinks do not promote life if they have sugar, high fructose corn syrup, or any artificial coloring. Tea has more caffeine than coffee. Caffeine is a diuretic of calcium and other minerals.

Chocolate milk contains a little-known chemical in the chocolate (also found in candy) called theo-bromine or methyl-xanthine. These chemicals disrupt brain function. Commercially manufactured milk shakes served at fast food restaurants normally contain plastic, chemical additives, and air. Fruit juices, consumed mostly by children, contain high fructose corn syrup and food coloring. Read labels on all beverages, including water. The ingredients should be natural—not artificial.

Natural Prescription for Health: Caffeine-free herbal teas are a logical alternative to coffee.

Personal Thoughts/Goals:

_____

_____

_____

_____

Day 20

Bethlehem Water

And David said with longing "Oh that someone would give me a drink of the water from the well of Bethlehem, which is by the gate!" (2 Samuel 23:15-17).

David's men risked their lives to retrieve water from Bethlehem. Imagine the sweet taste of water that Jesus consumed at Jacob's well. Who would have thought there would be a point in our lives when we would be searching for pure sources of water?

Water with microscopic particles, whether organic from the soil or inorganic from a human-made substance, creates unnecessary stress on our body's very sensitive kidney water filtration system. I have noticed that patients who do not drink water, but prefer soda consumption, tend to have kidney stone issues. If you suspect kidney irritation, there is a simple test. Have someone place the palm of the hand over your lower mid-back and gently but firmly apply pressure. If the test causes pain and the pain persists, you need to be evaluated by a healthcare provider.

Natural Prescription for Health: Avoid water that is not pleasant to the taste—it may contain harmful substances.

Personal Thoughts/Goals:

_____

_____

_____

_____

Day 21

Nibbles

In a Finnish study,[4] adults who regularly drank at least four cups of coffee a day had twice the risk of rheumatoid arthritis than those who drank less. In the early 1970s, when the study began, most Finns drank boiled coffee, so it's not clear whether filtered or decaffeinated coffee may also be linked to rheumatoid arthritis.

Women who consume more vitamin E-rich foods may have a lower risk of dying from a stroke, but it's not clear whether it's the vitamin E or something else in foods like nuts or full-fat salad dressings that may cut the risk.

> Previously I had constant pain in my back, right hip, and right knee along with depression, anxiety, and ADD. The information and care provided by Dr. DeMaria has improved my life. My pain is gone, and I have increased energy. The information that I receive encourages me to eat right and take vitamins and minerals. I started making changes to healthy, organic foods and drinking purified water (and more of it). I no longer eat junk food.
> —Wendy Johnson

Personal Thoughts/Goals:

_____

_____

_____

_____

Breath of Life Breakfast

Whatever Jesus did is relevant—including that He cooked breakfast for His disciples. The word *breakfast* means "breaking the fast." Think of your body as a furnace requiring fuel. My suggestion would be to put protein in your machine, which is similar to placing a slow-burning log or coal on a fire. Paper burns hot and quickly and needs to be replenished frequently, similar to fueling your body with pastry or doughnuts. Start every day with a protein or moderate glycemic index breakfast food.

As part of the last week of this pattern, you will have the opportunity to record your breakfast habits.

Eat breakfast for a healthy life.

Day 22

I Free You This Day

And now look, I free you this day from the chains that were on your hand…all the land [time] *is before you; wherever it seems good and convenient for you to go, go there* (Jeremiah 40:4).

You are free. You are free! Awesome words. Believers in Jesus are free from sin and death! Throw off the shackles of physical and emotional sickness. You have my permission—I am authorizing you with a renewed warranty of life. You would do best to follow natural, biblical health principles for the warranty to be intact. I know from experience that if you observe the following, you will live a happy and healthy life.

Because it is so important, here is another reminder to drink water daily from a pure source. Reverse osmosis is an excellent filter system. The following suggestions have been proven effective in maintaining optimal health: Eat primarily fresh organic vegetables, raw or steamed. Consume protein from an organic source. Focus on chicken, turkey, ocean fish, and lean red meat, but no pork. Consume one tablespoon of flax oil per one hundred pounds of body weight. Avoid refined sugar and all human-made substitutes. Never, ever eat trans fat or partially hydrogenated fat. Avoid liver-congesting beverages such as sugar-loaded sodas, fat-laden dairy products, and the substitute sugars found in diet sodas.

Ideally people should exercise a minimum of thirty minutes daily—weight training and aerobic. Meditate on God's Word constantly. Love everyone. Give to the poor. Have your spine checked for vertebral subluxation (dislocation of bone or joint). Meditate on the words of Jesus found in John 16:33.

Natural Prescription for Health: Make a quality decision to add one new health pattern to your life per day, week, or month. *Start now!*

Personal Thoughts/Goals:

_____

_____

_____

_____

Day 23

"Time for Breakfast!"

Jesus…took the bread and gave it to them, and likewise the fish (John 21:13).

"Come and eat breakfast," Jesus said to Peter after he caught 153 fish. I am sure Jesus was preparing Peter for his massive catch of souls shortly after eating this meal. Fish and fish oils, especially those derived from cold water sources, contain two important fats that are essential for bodily function—eicosapentaenoic acid (EPA) and docosahexaenoic acid (DHA). Salmon is a direct source of Omega 3 fat. Flax seeds and oil are plant precursors to Omega 3 fat.

The term *Omega 3* is the classification of fat required for blood vessel, heart, brain, and nerve health. Consuming this type of fat on a regular basis is an excellent way to prevent cardiovascular disease as well as emotional, memory, and behavioral disturbances.

Natural Prescription for Health: In the morning break the nighttime fast with hot water and lemon followed by fruit. One-half hour after digestive clearing of the fruit, enjoy protein (almonds, walnuts, pecans).

Personal Thoughts/Goals:

_____

_____

_____

_____

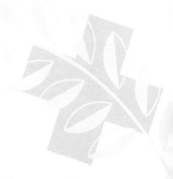

Day 24

Old Testament Food

…With the choicest wheat… (Deuteronomy 32:14).

One of the main obstacles to overcome is knowing what to eat or what not to eat to achieve optimal health. Confusion is easily created by reading what different experts recommend—one person's passion is another's poison.

Old Testament food *was not* genetically altered to resist pests. Food today has been *modified* to enhance the resistance caused by the elements or to create larger sizes without the inconvenience of seeds in fruits and vegetables. The Bible specifically states in Genesis 1:11, "*The herb that yields seed,*" not mutated or seedless—what a thought! Seeds are a life source. To eliminate them is to limit life or the reproduction of life.

Grain products are altered in the milling process. Avoiding bleached-enriched foods promotes life. Refining flour depletes the vitamins and minerals necessary for energy. Many breakfast cereals contain sugar, hydrogenated or trans fat, and preservatives that are depleted of essential vitamins and minerals. I encourage my patients to use rice, almond, or coconut milk on organic cereals if this is their choice of breakfast.

Gluten grains are a common cause of allergies and pain and even sleep apnea. Rotate your grains to include quinoa, brown rice, millet, and amaranth.

Natural Prescription for Health: Focus on organic, no GMO foods. GMO foods are those that are genetically modified. You will start to see NO GMO on food labels. Certified organic foods do not contain GMO ingredients. Try breads other than wheat—spelt grain items are available in most grocery stores.

Personal Thoughts/Goals:

_____

_____

_____

_____

Day 25

Gas Pedal

While the earth remains, seedtime and harvest, cold and heat,
winter and summer, and day and night shall not cease (Genesis 8:22).

Imagine your body is like a machine. The liver is the oil filter, the lungs are the muffler, the brain is the electric circuit, and your thyroid is the gas pedal. Every vehicle has a maintenance schedule, warranty, and operator's manual. The Bible is our manual. Read, follow, and observe the schedule, and you will enjoy a healthy life journey and be capable of navigating the peaks and valleys. Abuse your machine and you will end up on the junk heap prematurely.

The thyroid helps the body adjust to hot and cold. Does the initial cold of winter penetrate your bones? If so, the thyroid may need a more quality source of iodine. We suggest Celtic Sea Salt, organic kelp, sea vegetables found in the macrobiotic section of select grocery and health food stores, and organic iodine. Also, the liver needs to be functioning optimally to process oils, proteins, and hormones for thyroid use.

You can check the thyroid by monitoring your morning armpit temperature for three consecutive days. Take it first thing in the morning before you get out of bed. It should be 97.8 degrees or higher. Signs of low thyroid include constipation, morning headaches, wide-spaced teeth, fatigue throughout the day, and elevated cholesterol.

Natural Prescription for Health: Add Celtic Sea Salt to your food. It is not sodium chloride or table salt. It is a pure, non-altered natural mineral source.

Personal Thoughts/Goals:

_____

_____

_____

_____

Day 26

Juice and Fiber

Like an apple tree among the trees of the woods, so is my beloved among the sons.
I sat down in his shade with great delight, and his fruit was sweet to my taste
(Song of Solomon 2:3).

Fresh fruits and vegetables add enormous benefits to the human machine. Always think "living food" versus canned, frozen, or commercially prepared, vacuumed food and drink. Fresh rules! A special note: Food (that is not organic) on conventional store shelves is often picked before it ripens naturally and has been gassed, sprayed, and waxed to enhance appearance. I prefer patients eat fresh, organic vegetables and fruits. The fiber is necessary to cleanse the colon. You also lower cholesterol by eating fiber because it gently scrapes and brushes the mineral-absorbing intestinal villi.

I discourage drinking any carton or canned juices that have been pasteurized or concentrated. You want fresh, whole juice with nothing artificial added. Oxygen combines with vitamin C in juices to make it ineffective in a short time. Read the ingredients on all cans or containers. Avoid high fructose corn syrup, sodium benzoate (a preservative that causes allergies), and any added colors. These chemicals cause stress on your liver and kidneys where all toxins are cleaned out.

Natural Prescription for Health: The natural juice formula I recommend includes drinking eight ounces of fresh, organic ingredients: beet, carrot, celery, apple, parsley, cucumber, and a small piece of ginger. Obtain a durable juicer to make fresh juice daily. I use the Acme brand.

Personal Thoughts/Goals:

_____

_____

_____

Day 27

Test the Heart

The words of his mouth were smoother than cream or butter, but war was in his heart; his words were softer than oil, yet they were drawn swords (Psalm 55:21 AMP).

Jesus let the people know that He not only needed the words of their mouth—He really wanted their hearts. Words can be smooth as cream or butter. Cream is a dairy product that goes down with ease and can create pain because it is made of a fat called arachidonic acid. Dairy consumption may lead to pain in the body.

Butter, on the other hand, is neither good nor bad, but neutral. Butter can be used to sauté since it can be warmed to high temperatures. It is better than margarine but don't use too much.

Words have also been described to be softer than oil. I alert my patients about oils that they put *in* and *on* their bodies. Sodium Laurate (a toxic substance) in cosmetic oils and lotions can be easily absorbed by the lymph system, congesting the lymph system and impairing liver function.

To promote life: Drink and absorb fresh, clean water. Allow the words of your mouth to parallel the emotions of your heart—kind, uplifting words.

Natural Prescription for Health: Sauté eggs, spinach, and mushrooms in butter for breakfast. Skip the margarine.

Personal Thoughts/Goals:

_____

_____

_____

_____

Day 28

The Best Diet

People who eat a healthy diet—according to the "Alternate Healthy Eating Index"[5] created by Harvard University researchers—have a ten to twenty percent lower risk of disease (and a thirty to forty percent lower risk of heart disease) than people who eat a poor diet. The Harvard index is based on following more than one hundred thousand people for eight to twelve years.

The advice in the "Alternate Healthy Eating Index" should come as no surprise. Here's what people with the highest scores averaged:

- **Vegetables:** five servings a day

- **Fruit:** four servings a day

- **Fiber from cereals, breads, and grains:** nine grams a day (men) and seven grams a day (women)

- **Red meat:** six times (men) or three times (women) *more fish and poultry* than beef, pork, and lamb

- **Saturated fat:** thirty to forty percent less saturated fat than poly-unsaturated fat

- **Nuts:** one serving a day.

- **Multivitamins:** forty-five percent (men) or twenty-seven percent (women) had been taking a multivitamin for more than five years

Natural Prescription for Health: The Harvard diet advice is logical, with one qualification. If you don't drink alcohol, don't start now. Alcohol abuse contributes to traffic accidents, drownings, falls, industrial accidents, homicides, suicides, and spousal and child abuse.[6]

When I first came to see Dr. DeMaria, I had migraines, back pain, and neck pain. I was on four different kinds of medications. The information provided by Dr. Bob has improved my life for the better. I have modified my diet and try to eat more fruit. —Margaret Gutwein

Personal Thoughts/Goals:

_____

_____

_____

_____

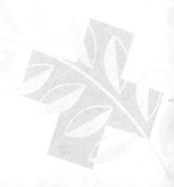

Day 29

You Are Known by Your Fruit

Every good tree bears good fruit but a bad tree bears bad fruit. A good tree cannot bear bad fruit, nor can a bad tree bear good fruit (Matthew 7:17-18).

Someone who is strong, healthy, happy, and fun to be around attracts your attention. That person is a joy to be with. Do you have people in your life who you try to avoid? Do people avoid you? This may be a wake-up call!

Fruit consumption restores important nutrients in the body. Fruit is a great source of fiber, especially the apple, which is necessary to keep your bowels functioning regularly. Blueberries are one of the best antioxidant foods. Antioxidants are like rustproof paint. They take the brown off of freshly cut apples.

Fructose, which is fruit sugar, not to be confused with high fructose corn syrup (HFCS), does not stress the pancreas like white table sugar. Eating fruit can help restore needed nutrients and improve bowel function, all which are needed to live a happy life! Some fruit, though, should be eaten in moderation. Patients who suffer with left neck and mid-back pain may have a common source for that pain—the regular consumption of bananas, raisins, grapes, pineapple, and any dried fruit. All of these fruits are loaded with sugar.

Natural Prescription for Health: Peel and dice fresh apple pieces and simmer over medium heat. Add cinnamon, chill, and enjoy a fresh applesauce treat!

Personal Thoughts/Goals:

_____

_____

_____

_____

Day 30

Dr. Bob's ABCs for Life

He causes…vegetation for the service of man… (Psalm 104:14).

It all started in the Garden of Eden. There were fruit trees, plants, and herbs to sustain life. However, current trends in time and family meal management focus on convenience at the expense of the natural quality of enhancing nutrients. Our bodies have had to make do with what they have been fed, leaving our bodies to figure out how to eliminate the toxic residue.

As a part of my patient coaching workshops, I encourage the following daily protocol. You should eat half of an apple daily. The **a**pple has malic acid to help thin bile for better digestion as well as fiber and pectin for bulk and healing. Wash and eat the peel along with the seeds. **B**eets and their fiber, especially grated raw, organic, act as an intestinal wall cleanser. Pickled and canned beets should be your last choice. **C**arrots have vitamin A for skin, eye, and liver health. Raw, organic carrot slices or a handful of baby carrots go a long way in promoting basic body function.

Natural Prescription for Health: Apple for breakfast. Beets for lunch. Carrots for supper.

Personal Thoughts/Goals:

_____

_____

_____

_____

Day 31

Yogurt—Cause of Stealth Pain?

*Your lips, O my spouse, drip as the honeycomb; honey and **milk** are under your tongue...*
(Song of Solomon 4:11, emphasis added).

Paul said all things are lawful for us, but not necessarily good for us. Commercial, conventional American yogurt has permeated the breakfast and snack time market. People purchase yogurt for the calcium and protein it contains. The basic physiology is right on target, but let me share a few facts.

Read the label on the yogurt container. Sugar and high fructose corn syrup are added to satisfy people's sweet addiction. Pasteurization destroys the bacteria that people assume is benefiting their own natural intestinal flora. The casein, which is a protein in dairy products, is very difficult to digest and the "arachidonic" fat creates pain. This tip is especially for individuals with chronic sinus congestion. Your body uses your sinus cavities as a toxic release valve. Yogurt can also be the main cause of teenage acne.

Natural Prescription for Health: Sprinkle sesame seeds on your favorite dish for a source of calcium.

> I suffered from sinus headaches so badly that I eventually had to see a doctor for medical treatment to relieve the pain. I used to consume four to six sinus tablets plus three aspirins each day. The information and care provided to me from Dr. Bob encouraged me to change my eating habits, eliminating sugar from my diet. I have not had one sinus headache in over four years nor have I taken any sinus medication.
>
> I attribute this to my adjustments as well as my change in diet. By removing sugar, anyone's health would change for the better. —Dennis Skinner

Personal Thoughts/Goals:

_____

_____

_____

_____

Day 32

A Pink Toothbrush

*My God sent His angel and shut the lions' **mouths**…because I was found innocent before Him; and also, O king, I have done no wrong before you* (Daniel 6:22, emphasis added).

Is your bark bigger and stronger than your bite? The angel of the Lord kept the lions' teeth from chewing up Daniel in the den. Is the state of your teeth and gums preventing you from eating what your body needs for optimal health? There are several reasons why you may have a "pink toothbrush." A common cause today is gingivitis.

I know from experience that Americans get a limited amount of natural vitamin C complex from their diet. Lack of vitamin C can create weakness in teeth and gums resulting in fragile tissue and a pink toothbrush. I encourage patients to focus on bell peppers, which are an excellent source of complex C. Citrus may cause an alkaline pH as well as migrating muscle pain. Smoking depletes the body of precious vitamin C. I do not recommend eating chewable ascorbic acid as synthetic ascorbic acid does not promote long-term dental health. The acid is tough on the enamel.

Natural Prescription for Health: Do not chew synthetic vitamin C, ascorbic acid.

Personal Thoughts/Goals:

_____

_____

_____

_____

Day 33

Swine, Go Swimming

Now a large herd of swine was feeding there near the mountains....Then [with Jesus' permission] *the **unclean** spirits went out and entered the swine...and the herd ran violently down the steep place into the sea and drowned in the sea* (Mark 5:11,13, emphasis added).

Jesus asked the possessed man at Gadarenes how many unclean spirits there were. Then He proceeded to cast the unclean spirits into unclean animals. That was an enormous miracle. An interesting observation: A herd of two thousand swine was very valuable. The economic loss of the swine must have been alarming to the community.

Swine were and *still are* unclean animals. Pork *is not* the other white meat. Pork flesh, no matter how you cook it, is toxic. Question: Do you have a relentless thirst after eating ham? Reason: Your body is attempting to dilute toxins. Jesus, I believe, knew that pork was unclean—otherwise, why would He allow them to stampede to their death? Pass on the pork (especially pork sausage) the next time you are at a buffet or potluck. "No thank you" goes a long way to optimal health.

Natural Prescription for Health: Turkey bacon—from organic sources without nitrates and colors—is an alternative if you desire bacon and eggs.

Personal Thoughts/Goals:

_____

_____

_____

_____

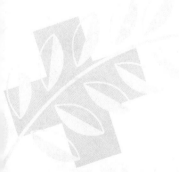

Day 34

What Shall We Eat?

...For your heavenly Father knows you need all these things (Matthew 6:32).

Food is an integral part of God's Word. Your body is required to work harder and can become stressed as it attempts to keep you functioning on dead, devitalized food. The pancreas is especially stressed by providing enzymes to properly break down "fake" food.

I encourage my patients to eat living food. Focus on food without labels. Canned, packaged, and vacuum-preserved foods have stickers describing the contents. Vegetables, fruits, whole grains, herbs eaten right from the vine or garden, along with fresh organic meat, poultry, or ocean fish that are steamed or broiled, promote life and require no labels.

Avoid all processed items.

Natural Prescription for Health: God-made food from seed-bearing, organic sources is the right choice. The strategy of label-savvy shoppers would be to look at the PLU number on your fruits and vegetables; the first number reveals the source—#9 indicates organic, #8 indicates genetically altered, and all other numbers indicate some type of additional chemical. An example of organic would be #97343; genetically engineered would be #86458.

Personal Thoughts/Goals:

_____

_____

_____

_____

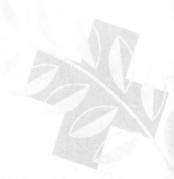

Day 35

Vitamin E & Eyes

Vitamin E supplements flunked a test to see if they could reduce the risk of macular degeneration, a common cause of blindness in older people. (The macula is the center of the retina.)

In an Australian study,[7] of one thousand healthy volunteers aged fifty-five to eighty, those who took five hundred IU of vitamin E every day for four years were no less likely to be diagnosed with macular degeneration than those who took a placebo (sugar pill).

Natural Prescription for Health: Until researchers know more about protecting eyesight, your safest bet is to eat a diet rich in fruits and vegetables, especially leafy greens.

Personal Thoughts/Goals:

_____

_____

_____

_____

Day 36

Is There Any Taste in the Egg White?

Can flavorless food be eaten without salt? Or is there any taste in the white of an egg?
(Job 6:6).

Eggs are one of the most complete foods on the planet, but we have lived in "egg phobia" for nearly thirty years. Eggs were discussed in God's Word in relation with salt. Can you believe it? Your body needs sodium. *Sodium* is an important mineral needed to reduce body stiffness and control allergies. But *sodium chloride* or "table salt" is an unhealthy combination. We suggest Celtic Sea Salt in our practice. It is pure, not whitened or chemically altered.

Eggs are not dairy. They are an excellent source of protein. Egg yolk has lecithin in it which helps emulsify the cholesterol. The best type of egg is a free range, high Omega-3 sourced, organic product, and it is best if fertilized. Eggs are also a quality source of sulfur. Sulfur is needed to make collagen and helps keep the phlegm in your throat tolerable and to a minimum. Contrary to accepted thought, eggs are not the main reason cholesterol is elevated in your body. An egg a day is healthier than a doughnut a day by far.

Eggs can be poached, basted, sunny-side-up, scrambled, or hard boiled. I prefer my eggs for breakfast. It is a good slow-burn fuel. Normally I scramble them in the morning with spinach.

Natural Prescription for Health: Add eggs to your diet regularly. Stay away from "plastic" liquid eggs in a carton.

Personal Thoughts/Goals:

_____

_____

_____

_____

Keeping a Breakfast Journal enables you to follow your progress as you journey toward more optimal health. You will use this information to complete the Self-Assessment Breakfast Debriefing at the end of this section.

Breakfast Journal:

_____

_____

_____

_____

Day 37

Melons—Fruit of the Vine

We remember the fish we ate freely in Egypt, the cucumbers, the melons...
(Numbers 11:5).

God created an inborn desire for sweets for survival. Human milk has a natural sweetness. But creating a sugar addiction in your infants and toddlers can cause a lifetime of health issues, so don't give your youngsters sugar or high fructose corn syrup.

Melons are an excellent source of minerals and vitamins, but limit your watermelon consumption. Watermelon has a high concentration of carbohydrates. I have seen patients have acute left neck and low back pain due to sugar overload from eating too much watermelon. Cantaloupe, on the other hand, is dense and lower in natural sugar than watermelon. Honeydew is somewhere between. Harvey Diamond, in his best seller *Fit for Life*, suggests eating melon first, prior to eating other fruit choices. A delicious "kid treat"—blend cantaloupe and honeydew in a food processor, separately, and pour the puree into ice cube trays for an afternoon refresher.

Natural Prescription for Health: Substitute a wedge of cucumber, a relative to the watermelon, for your potassium instead of a high-carbohydrate banana.

Personal Thoughts/Goals:

_____

_____

_____

_____

Breakfast Journal:

_____

_____

_____

_____

Day 38

A Whip for a Horse

A whip for a horse, a bridle for a donkey... (Proverbs 26:3).

Creating an optimal level of consistent health appears to be difficult to achieve for Western medical-thinking mindsets. Wellness or prevention is taking an aspirin for blood thinning or vaccination for the flu. If you owned a thoroughbred race horse, would you feed it fries, ice cream, soda, hot dogs, or food colorings? What do you feed yourself? Are you not more important than the sparrow? (See Matthew 10:31.) Feed your body whole food. Avoid deli meats; eat baked fries versus oil cooked; treat yourself to quality ice cream; and pass on the hot dogs.

The whip for a horse is similar to what a therapeutic herb does to the body. You can whip a poorly fed and trained race horse for a lap or two, but over time the animal will collapse. Likewise, do not feed yourself junk and expect an immune-boosting herb like Echinacea or a once-a-day synthetic multivitamin to rescue you.

Natural Prescription for Health: Start your day with food for a champion athlete: an egg and wholesome, fresh, organic almond butter on sprouted grain bread.

Personal Thoughts/Goals:

_____

_____

_____

_____

Breakfast Journal:

_____

_____

_____

_____

Day 39

"Bring to Remembrance"

…He [the Holy Spirit] *will teach you all things and bring to your remembrance all things that I said to you* (John 14:26).

God created our memory as a human secret weapon. The Holy Spirit came to us for several reasons—one is to tweak our memory.

You can increase your memory capacity. My first suggestion is to detoxify your body. I have seen patients who have toxic habits caused by a stressed liver due to a lifetime of poor food choices. These individuals have had thought lapses even in their twenties. Why does someone who works crossword puzzles and word games and reads and memorizes verses respond quickly when asked a question while those who watch hours and hours of TV answer with a blank stare? Start increasing your memory capacity by thinking and using your mind with activity versus being amused or entertained by TV and media.

Critical brain food for memory health is eating Omega 3 fat from plant sources. Low fat diets do not promote memory function.

Natural Prescription for Health: Shut off the TV today.

Personal Thoughts/Goals:

_____

_____

_____

_____

Breakfast Journal:

_____

_____

_____

_____

Day 40

Blueberries—Antioxidants

*...For why is my **liberty** judged by another man's conscience?*
(1 Corinthians 10:29, emphasis added).

Liberty: Freedom from external constraint.[8]

Prior to the Fall of Adam, all vegetation enjoyed timeless growth and liberty. Nature is seeking to be made free from the law of sin and death (see Rom. 8:2). Our bodies are in a constant state of breakdown and repair. Breakdown appears to occur with reckless abandonment while repair requires enormous energy.

Focus your daily activity to limit obvious damage from pollutants and toxins. While working at home or in the yard, it is prudent to follow directions to keep skin, lungs, and clothing from being exposed to hazardous chemicals. You can promote cellular health and protection by choosing foods that act as natural barriers to toxins similar to a clear coat of wax on motor vehicles.

One of the best antioxidant choices that protects the body from oxygenated chemical reactions is blueberries. Regular consumption of blueberries promotes life. Remember, fruit is best eaten alone followed by some type of nut protein.

Natural Prescription for Health: Always consider fresh vegetables and fruit in your daily schedule of food choices. Blueberries and spinach are at the top of the list.

Personal Thoughts/Goals:

_____

_____

_____

Breakfast Journal:

_____

_____

_____

Day 41

Dr. Bob's Breakfast

Jesus said to them, "Come down and eat breakfast" (John 21:12 paraphrased).

What is the breakfast of champions? What do you feed yourself? I normally start my day with hot water and lemon. I make half-caffeine, half-decaffeinated organic coffee with organic cream. On work days, I eat two scrambled eggs with spinach and mushrooms. I use butter or olive oil. No bread; I try to minimize bread. I do eat it, but not regularly. I do not eat pancakes or waffles. I eat tomatoes, carrots, and half an apple around 10:00 or 10:30 a.m. as a midmorning snack.

On days when I have the morning off, I consume half an apple with nuts, usually almonds, for breakfast. I do not start my day with a lot of fruit, avoiding bananas, grapes, and raisins. Occasionally, I eat oatmeal with almonds, flax seeds, or shredded coconut. It's always tasty to add applesauce if we have a fresh homemade batch available. If I eat a bagel or English muffin, I have almond butter or olive oil on it. Avoid foods that elevate insulin like breakfast cereals.

Natural Prescription for Health: Focus on medium or low glycemic index food for breakfast—choose protein.

Personal Thoughts/Goals:

_____

_____

_____

_____

Breakfast Journal:

_____

_____

_____

_____

Day 42

Fruit and Veggie Diet

Can a diet rich in fruits and vegetables keep you trim? Nutritionists say yes, and now there's data to back them up.

Researchers tracked more than 74,000 women aged thirty-eight to sixty-three for twelve years. Those who *boosted* their intake of fruits and vegetables by four servings a day had a twenty-four percent lower risk of obesity than those who *cut* their fruits and vegetables by about two servings a day.[9]

Natural Prescription for Health: Pack some baby carrots for snacks, start breakfast with wedges of cantaloupe, serve at least two vegetables for dinner. Who can complain about roasted asparagus, broccoli in garlic sauce, or sautéed spinach?

> I came to see Dr. DeMaria because I had bad acne, sinus infections, stiff neck, headaches, fluid in my ears, and allergy attacks. I was taking medication for my sinuses, which I don't need much anymore. Following Dr.'s recommendations, I have eliminated sugar and dairy, and I now eat more green veggies and drink more water. I feel much better every day. I know that my healing process is well on its way. God made us; He knows how to fix us. But it is a process and requires discipline. Thank God for the knowledge that He has given to Dr. Bob. —Nia Greenhill

Personal Thoughts/Goals:

_____

_____

_____

_____

Self-Assessment
Breakfast Debriefing

Using the information you wrote in your Breakfast Journals, answer the following questions and mark your score as directed. Your goal is a score of five.

_____ Did you eat breakfast each day? Add one.

_____ Did you focus on proteins, egg, oatmeal with almonds, beans, almond butter, fish, and animal or plant protein? Add one.

_____ What beverage did you have? Water, water with lemon, herbal tea, fresh-made vegetable juice? Add one. Coffee, decaf or regular, soda, commercial fruit or vegetable juice, milk or dairy product, caffeine tea? Subtract one.

_____ Did you have a refined wheat grain, pastry, Danish, doughnut, bagel, muffin? Subtract one.

_____ Did you have a sprouted grain product? Add one.

_____ Did you have a fresh, in-season fruit? Add one.

_____ Did you eat at home? Add one.

_____ Did you eat on the run in a car, plane, or train? Subtract one.

_____ Did you use a sugar substitute? Subtract one.

_____ Did you eat margarine? Subtract one.

_____ Did you use butter? No change.

_____ Did you use olive or flax oil? Add one.

_____ Did you have animal protein with starch (meat and potatoes)? Subtract one.

_____ Did you have organic almonds, walnuts, pecans, or cashews? Add one.

_____ Total score

Dr. Bob's breakfast comment: Your goal is to eat a meal in the morning. Eat low or mid-glycemic food. A great example would be oatmeal with almonds, with a glycemic number of 78; or you could try some barley, which has an index number of 36. Combine foods accurately. My clinical experience suggests wheat-based products may be the cause of pain in some patients.

I would like to encourage you to become a student in the ever-changing category of food products on the grocer's shelves. Genetically-engineered products are showing up on the grocery baskets of uninformed consumers. Items you once purchased from a health food–based company now may have new owners who are concerned about the bottom line with increased profits.

There are several categories of food groups that were once considered healthy and excellent for promoting optimal health that now are major causative saboteurs. I would like you to be aware that the night shaded food group may create pain and distress in your body; tomatoes, white potatoes, green peppers, hot peppers, eggplant and paprika are the most common. The impact of this group has accelerated from my observation because so many today have compromised liver function. The liver is overwhelmed by an alkaloid toxin called solanine, which is a known stressor.

Gluten is a protein found in wheat, rye, oats, and, barley. Gluten may impair absorption of nutrients in your colon and actually be a cause of heart palpitations, digestive distress, bloating, and even anemia. Forty-one percent of people in the US have the gene for celiac disease, but only one percent manifest symptoms of the condition— painful colon function and malabsorption syndrome with loose stools. I have discovered that the gluten in many products may create an almost immediate reaction in some people; others may not even realize that the way they feel is caused by some of their favorite pastries, breads, and cereals. Adding B6 at 150 milligrams a day, two teaspoons of Omega 3 liquid anchovy/sardine based oil magnesium, and a full spectrum protein may help. I would encourage you to seek the advice of a skilled healthcare provider.

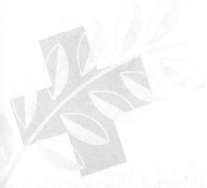

Energizing Exercise

Jesus walked to many places during His ministry. He must have been physically fit to carry the heavy cross to Golgotha (see John 19). He endured much. Focus on alternating aerobics such as walking, running, tennis, racquet ball, or biking, along with muscle toning exercises that include free weights, bands, and fitness machines. Regular exercise improves posture, fluid movement, and "feel good" hormones called endorphins. For optimal health, exercise a minimum of three times to five times weekly. I encourage my patients to exercise thirty minutes at a time. There are twenty-four hours in every day; thirty minutes is a very short time, considering the positive impact.

Day 43

Exercise for Life

And everyone who competes for the prize is temperate in all things. Now they do it to obtain a perishable crown, but we for an imperishable crown. Therefore I run thus: not with uncertainty. Thus I fight: not as one who beats the air. But I discipline my body and bring it into subjection, lest, when I have preached to others, I myself should become disqualified (1 Corinthians 9:25-27).

Regular exercise promotes efficient burning of blood sugar. Muscles need fuel to perform their purpose. You can help control your blood glucose by simple activities, including walking, bike riding, and jogging. Experts suggest that walking ten thousand steps daily, or about five miles, will help burn off some extra calories you have consumed. Each mile is about 2,500 steps. It takes 7,990 steps to burn off the average cheeseburger. Doughnuts take 5,750 steps; a 12-ounce can of soda takes 3,450 steps; a garden salad with fat-free dressing takes 1,160 steps.

Wear arch-supporting walking shoes and drink plenty of water. Cramping while walking may be a sign of a mineral need or lack of proper blood flow.

Natural Prescription for Health: Choose a regular activity with motion. Ships in the harbor attract rust and barnacles. Don't go down with the ship! Keep moving!

Personal Thoughts/Goals:

_____

_____

_____

_____

Day 44

Building Muscle Strength

...And works it with the strength of his arms... (Isaiah 44:12).

A common dilemma as we mature is loss of muscle firmness and strength. It is true that "you lose what you don't use." Muscle strength breakdown can result in a very huge negative issue. Your body uses muscle to burn extra glucose you don't need from eating more than you should. Poor metabolism of carbohydrates, especially refined grains and sugar in pasta, white bread, muffins, Danish, bagels, and so forth, depletes the body of zinc. Low zinc levels reduce insulin output. Your body needs fuel in the cells brought in by the insulin. Without energy from the carbohydrate mechanism, your body systems use protein taken from muscle. Over time, reducing muscle mass results in a catch-22 with more unused carbs continuing to metabolize to fat.

I would recommend that you reduce refined carbohydrate intake and start light to moderate muscle strengthening. Using handheld weights and elastic bands is a great way to begin.

Natural Prescription for Health: Light resistance training with weights or elastic bands promotes solid bone integrity. Start today.

Personal Thoughts/Goals:

_____

_____

_____

_____

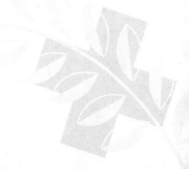

Day 45

Obesity Epidemic

You shall eat, but not be satisfied… (Micah 6:14).

"*My people are destroyed for lack of knowledge*" (Hos. 4:6). Manufacturers are required by the law to list product ingredients. To reach your goal of optimal health, you must obtain nutrition knowledge and become a label reader; don't be ignorant of the facts.

There are foods, additives, and sweeteners that fly below the radar screen of the consumer's consciousness. The most prevalent is high fructose corn syrup. When you break the word down, fructose is fruit sugar. But corn is good for you, and syrup comes from maple trees, right? *Wrong!* High fructose corn syrup (HFCS) has permeated nearly every item you purchase today that has a label on it. You can even find HFCS in chocolate milk. We have become a society that craves sweetness.

Unfortunately, the calories consumed with this type of human-made fractionalized fructose do not trigger the normal feed backloop in the eating cycle. When you eat HFCS, you will still be hungry, even to the last bite. You will eat and drink and still be thirsty and hungry—increasing your weight with each bite and sip! The manufacturers know this—now you do too.

Natural Prescription for Health: Avoid food with high fructose corn syrup, which tends to reduce the hormone leptin, which tells your brain you are full. It is possible to be hungry after you drink a HFCS beverage or food; for example, having applesauce, which is "healthy," but is sweetened with HFCS, can alter your natural desire for food.

Personal Thoughts/Goals:

_____

_____

_____

_____

Day 46

Cravings

And the world passes away and disappears, and with it the forbidden cravings…
(1 John 2:17 AMP).

Ultimately, craving a deep relationship with the Lord will satisfy all your worldly desires. However, forbidden cravings or addictions result in a very poor state of health.

The most common craving I help patients overcome is the addiction to sugar. Sugar robs the body of minerals and vitamins. Once the cycle is started, it is hardly different than being addicted to drugs, including alcohol. I believe sugar and its negative effects are from the devil. The devil came to steal, kill, and destroy.

I encourage my patients to increase their protein consumption during the day. Nuts, chicken, and turkey are great sources of protein. Chromium levels are often low in individuals desiring sugar. Sometimes a coating of fat can surround cell membranes, preventing your body from accessing badly needed glucose. I suggest a natural bile salt supplement with meals.

Natural Prescription for Health: Increase protein, which will stop the craving for carbohydrates and reduce blood pressure.

Personal Thoughts/Goals:

_____

_____

_____

_____

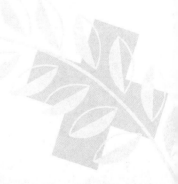

Day 47

Cornerstone Significance

Having been built on the foundation of the apostles and prophets,
Jesus Christ Himself being the chief cornerstone (Ephesians 2:20).

Jesus is our cornerstone. A cornerstone is the point of the building where two significant walls join. In biblical terms, this is the primary focal point of "the spiritual person" and "the physical person." Jesus unites the Bride and Groom. Each one of us who have accepted Jesus as our personal Savior is analogous to a brick in the Church. Masonry bricks make strong structures. They can last for decades without continuous maintenance. When my family was in Jericho, we asked the guide what happened to the stones that made the walls of Jericho. She responded that the neighboring inhabitants came and took them. The neighbors knew the strong nature of those building bricks.

The cornerstone in your body frame is the spine. We don't think much about the spine since we cannot see it, like our teeth. For optimal health, we need to focus on standing and sitting erect. Here is a tip. When standing, focus on holding your shoulders back. I encourage my patients to grasp their hands and place them in the small of their back. This will naturally position your shoulders behind a forward head alignment. Spinal breakdown is effortless—erect posture requires energy.

Natural Prescription for Health: Look at your posture in the mirror. *I generally see elevated left shoulders on patients who eat sugar.* How is your shoulder elevation? You can check for techno neck—forward head posture from using your phone, video games, and computers. Have someone take a digital side posture of you standing in your natural stance. Your ear should be over the middle of your shoulder. Every inch your ear is forward increases the weight of your head by ten pounds.

Personal Thoughts/Goals:

_____

_____

_____

_____

Day 48

Sunning

…Because the sun has tanned me… (Song of Solomon 1:6).

God put the sun in the sky to provide light for up to sixteen hours a day. The sun's rays are a part of a healthy wellness plan. Sunlight converts the cholesterol in your skin to vitamin D, which is needed for calcium absorption.

Do you ever notice how many people have lip cold sores after returning home from a sunny winter trip? The sun used up their calcium reserves. Cold sores on the lip can be caused by lack of calcium. I encourage my patients to consume additional flax oil and calcium citrate when they will be in the sun more than usual.

You can diminish sun damage by limiting or eliminating trans fat or partially hydrogenated fats. Protecting your skin with a lotion that has natural, non-petrochemical ingredients is logical. I warn my patients against applying baby oils on the skin because commercial oils may plug the lymph system.

Natural Prescription for Health: Walk in the early morning or early evening sun.

Personal Thoughts/Goals:

_____

_____

_____

_____

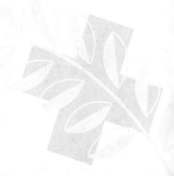

Day 49

Syndrome X

One out of five Americans have the metabolic syndrome, a national survey reports.[10] Among people in their sixties or seventies, the rate is two out of five. Also known as Syndrome X, the metabolic syndrome is a cluster of abnormalities that raise the risk of heart disease. You have it if you have at least three of the following:

- Blood pressure of at least 130 (systolic) or at least 85 (diastolic)

- Fasting blood sugar of at least 110

- Triglycerides of at least 150

- HDL (good) cholesterol of less than 40 (men) or less than 50 (women)

- A waist measurement of at least 35 inches (women) or at least 40 inches (men)

Natural Prescription for Health: Exercise (even if you don't lose weight) and weight loss (even if you don't lose much) can reverse the metabolic syndrome. Replacing carbohydrates (like sweets, bread, and pasta) with small quantities of unsaturated fats (from nuts, oils, and salad dressing) may also help. If you have even one of the metabolic syndrome's five risk factors, put down the soft drink can and get off your duff. The older you get, the closer you'll be to having at least three of these symptoms.

> Before I made Dr. DeMaria's recommended lifestyle changes, I was suffering with TMJ pain, pain in my arms, occasional back pain, digestive problems, and seasonal depression that was encouraged by pain. Following Dr.'s advice, I began to exercise, stopped drinking milk and coffee, started eating more organic foods when possible, and began taking recommended vitamins, flax oil, and salmon oil. It has been difficult to change my schedule to allow time for exercise. I no longer take Vioxx and Wellbutrin. I am now much better able to handle the "winter blues" without pain. I feel pretty much pain free. I feel much better about not taking medications and hope to limit my use of prescription medications. —Karen Netherland

Personal Thoughts/Goals:

_____

_____

_____

_____

Day 50

Stand Tall

*Put on the whole armor of God, that you may **stand** against the wiles of the devil*
(Ephesians 6:11, emphasis added).

Look at your posture; others do. Is your trunk in a forward position? Are your shoulders round? The "Doorjamb Push-up" will help stabilize your trunk position and vitalize your lung capacity. Forward postures generally result in poor health.

The Doorjamb Push-up is a simple maneuver designed to pull the shoulders back. A forward head position is not a healthy posture alignment.

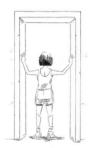 Stand in the middle of a doorway (see figure). Raise your hands to shoulder height or above, place the palms on the doorjamb, and lean your body into the doorway. Remain in this position for five seconds. Do this exercise daily—three sets of fifteen.

Natural Prescription for Health: Daily Doorjamb Push-ups relieve mid-back pain and prevent "round back."

Personal Thoughts/Goals:

_____

_____

_____

_____

Day 51

Stand for Truth

Stand therefore, having girded your waist with truth, having put on the breastplate of righteousness (Ephesians 6:14).

Your posture is the window to your nervous system. A forward head position is one of the most challenging to slow, stop, and reverse. Take your time with incorporating this exercise into your daily routine; it may cause initial lower neck pain, which will go away.

This exercise requires a weight bench, picnic table bench, or a coffee table. While lying on your back, slide your head/trunk to the end of your support structure. Slide off until you are mid-shoulder blade or lower. Hang your head, shoulders, and upper trunk off the edge (see figure). Remain in this position for about thirty seconds. Increase your time up to two minutes daily. This is an excellent active maneuver, which strengthens the trunk and pulls the upper body backward. Forward body posture puts a pull on the brain, spinal cord, and spinal nerves.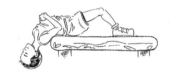

Natural Prescription for Health: Hand, arm, and wrist pain can diminish with this maneuver. Place a "fluffy" paint roller in the back of your neck for additional curve support.

Personal Thoughts/Goals:

_____

_____

_____

_____

Day 52

Stand Against Evil

*Therefore, take up the whole armor of God, that you may be able to withstand
in the evil day, and having done all, to stand* (Ephesians 6:13).

An optimal functioning spine means an optimal functioning nervous system which means optimal health. When your head is in a forward position, your brain can literally be pulled into your skull floor. Gravity relentlessly pushes you down. You can slow the destructive compression of gravity with the following exercise.

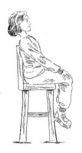

The head glide takes some concentration (see figure). Sit with your eyes closed. Slide your head and upper neck straight backward, then tilt chin up slightly. Do not move your shoulders. This is an excellent way to establish and maintain a normal cervical curve. A normal lordotic cervical curve will increase the strength of your spine by a factor of seven. Hold the head position for five seconds. Complete three sets of 15 every day. You may feel slight neck pain at first, but this exercise will prevent long-term spinal imbalance and will help minimize the damage caused by subluxation once your subluxations are checked and corrected. (See Day 288 for a more detailed explanation of subluxation.)

Natural Prescription for Health: Your eyeglasses position may need to be adjusted with this maneuver. Eliminate bananas, raisins, grapes, and any dried fruit to relieve left neck pain.

Personal Thoughts/Goals:

_____

_____

_____

_____

Day 53

Mental Contentment

Not that I speak in regard to need, for I have learned in whatever state I am,
to be content... (Philippians 4:11).

Love, joy and peace—fruits of the spirit—are precursors for mental peace. We live in an information-driven and media-driven society where everything from morning razor blades to evening dinner containers are disposable. Paul was content in all things. How can you be content when being constantly bombarded with product advertisements promising to make you feel better, look better, clean better, and so forth? A couple of tips: Before you go grocery shopping, make a list and buy only what is on the list. Also, do not go into the store if you are feeling hungry. These two steps will help control spontaneous spending.

Mental confusion, mental instability, or noises in the head can be a sign of whole food B vitamin deficiency. One of the most common underlying causes of many conditions I assess is the B-complex deficiency syndrome. Having constant noises and emotional turmoil can create chaos and drain you emotionally. Self-inflicted, negative self-talk can also deplete necessary B-vitamins. Sugar is by far the leading cause of B vitamin deficiency.

Natural Prescription for Health: Do you cry without reason or crave sugar? Add whole-grain B vitamin food to your meals. Oats, rye, millet, spelt, barley, and brown rice are excellent sources.

Personal Thoughts/Goals:

_____

_____

_____

_____

Day 54

A Bit of History—Step Climbing

Then they led Jesus from Caiaphas to the Praetorium, and it was early morning...
Pilate then went out to them... (Matthew 11:27, 29).

Martin Luther, German theologian and leader of the Reformation, was impacted by his step-climbing experience at the Santa Scala in Rome. Martin Luther was there to pay penance for his grandfather's soul in purgatory. I had an opportunity to walk those same steps. It is believed that Jesus walked these steps while being questioned by Pilate at the time of His crucifixion. Centuries later, the Praetorium steps were taken by Constantine's mother as a war souvenir. Religious tradition and indulgences, still observed by many today, were part of Luther's motivation to write his thesis in 1517.

Stair climbing, in the natural, is an excellent cardiovascular exercise for your heart and lungs. I encourage my patients to walk regularly. A stair-step machine is a valuable piece of equipment that strengthens your butt muscles and supports your spine and thigh muscles and will even tighten up painful weak knees.

Natural Prescription for Health: Walk up the steps instead of using the escalator or elevator. You will reduce pain and improve back and knee strength.

Personal Thoughts/Goals:

_____

_____

_____

_____

Day 55

Knowledge and Passion

For God so loved the world that He gave His only begotten Son... (John 3:16).

Knowledge is power. Application of knowledge is wisdom. Passion blended with knowledge is the foundation for an extraordinary life. Jesus had passion for His purpose. He was relentless in His pursuit to go to the Cross, even to the point of rebuking Peter and telling him to get behind Him.

In my practice, I see patients who do not have knowledge as to how the body functions. Always remember that the food you eat becomes you. Hot dogs, bologna, fries, and soda become your nerves, eyes, hair, blood, and emotional state. People have challenges getting passionate when they are not one hundred percent healthy. Fatigue, common in Americans, prevents focusing for long time periods. Regular exercise diminishes depression without the need for medications. More energy is another benefit.

Sugar fogs the mind and memory. Lack of sleep slows sharpness in decisions. Exercise, by far, is the one activity that will do a lot for increasing your energy and thinking capabilities. Start some form of regular exercise. Find a specific area in God's Word on which you can meditate to increase God's Kingdom. Seek the Lord for your purpose, and turn up your passion a notch.

Natural Prescription for Health: *Read* God's Word. *Chew* on what you read. *Act* on what the Lord is telling you to do.

Personal Thoughts/Goals:

_____

_____

_____

_____

Day 56

Diabetes: Zero Risk

Middle-aged women who exercise, eat a healthy diet, don't smoke, and—most importantly—aren't overweight can virtually eliminate their risk of diabetes.

Some specifics: Women who are overweight are eight times more likely to be diagnosed with the disease than lean women. Obese women are twenty times more likely.

Women who engage in at least seven hours a week of brisk walking, heavy gardening or housework, or other activities "vigorous enough to build up a sweat" have a thirty percent lower risk than women who exercise less than half an hour a week.

Women who eat the most high-fiber cereals and breads (rather than sweets, potatoes, and other refined carbohydrates) and the most polyunsaturated fats (rather than saturated and *trans* fats) have half the risk.[11]

Natural Prescription for Health: Cut back on hamburgers, pizza, fries, ice cream, and sweets. Replace them with beans, fish, whole-grain breads, cereals, fruits, vegetables, and (if you can afford the calories) salad dressings and vegetable oils. Watch your weight and don't forget: Exercise cuts the risk of diabetes even if you never lose a pound. I would also recommend you have your healthcare provider request an A1C, which is the glucose on a red blood cell; this is an excellent screen to help you determine your blood sugar status. Elevated A1C levels are a signal for you to cut back on refined sugar and grains and to get moving to burn the extra glucose molecules.

> When I began care with Dr. DeMaria, I had very high cholesterol. My "conventional thinking" doctor wanted to start me on Lipitor. After reading about this drug and the side effects, I decided to try something else. I have cut way back on sugar, and I don't go close to vending machines—no pop or soda. I have also started the ABC's to health—apples, beets, and carrots. It has been difficult reducing my sugar intake; no pies, cakes, or junk food, including chips, Tostitos, and Doritos. Since following Dr. Bob's advice, I have lowered my cholesterol some 20 points and lowered my triglycerides 170 points. I also have no aches or pains like I did before. —Fred Smith

Personal Thoughts/Goals:

_____

_____

Day 57

Steps to Restore Health

For I will restore health to you... (Jeremiah 30:17).

So where do you start the process of health restoration? You need to make a covenant with God that you will make the decision to see yourself healthy. Always be aware of what you say about your condition. You become what you speak. Socialize with happy, healthy, cheerful people. Avoid negative encounters.

Focus on living food versus processed, overcooked, and chemically altered "wannabe" foods. Clean machines work better—drink water from a pure source. Start your day with a minimum of one measured quart bottle as a part of your wardrobe. Begin a regular "oxygen stimulating" exercise routine such as aerobics, walking, weight training, elastic bands, machines, or hand weights. Exercise keeps the frame toned and solid. Sleep a minimum of six to eight hours nightly. Getting to sleep before midnight is life-enhancing. You do not want to depend on your "second wind"—your immune system will be stressed.

Read Scripture out loud daily. God did not *think* light to Himself. He *said*, "Let there be light." Forgive everyone; love your neighbor as yourself!

Natural Prescription for Health: Eat fresh (not canned), fiber-rich food (such as beans, broccoli, cabbage, and vegetables) to promote colon movement.

Personal Thoughts/Goals:

_____

_____

_____

_____

Day 58

Foot Gear

And he preached, saying, "There comes One after me who is mightier than I, whose sandal strap I am not worthy to stoop down and loose" (Mark 1:7).

Proper foot gear is a necessity if you don't want bunions, hammer toes, and calluses. John the Baptist said he was not worthy to even unlace the thong or latchet of Jesus' sandal. The sandal of the chosen people lasted forty years. When God makes something, He does it right.

Here's a thought. If you daily spend a full eight to ten hours on your feet—change your shoes halfway through the day. Your feet will thank you. I regularly change shoes since I am on my feet for extended periods of time. Dress for comfort. High-heeled shoes can create a painful dropped foot bone called a metatarsal. There is also a condition called Tarsal Tunnel, which creates pain on the inside of the ankle. Jogging or running shoes can wear out and cause knee, ankle, hip, and back pain. Shoes that are old and worn out should be replaced.

The following exercise will help promote quality, long-term foot mechanics. While sitting with feet straight ahead and flat on the floor, raise your toes up and down slowly for twenty-five repetitions, holding for a count of five. Turn your feet outward and repeat. Turn your feet inward and repeat.

Natural Prescription for Health: Schedule a pedicure periodically to maintain foot wellness.

Personal Thoughts/Goals:

_____

_____

_____

_____

Day 59

John and Peter Ran

*So they both ran together and the other disciple **outran** Peter and came to the tomb first*
(John 20:4 emphasis added).

What an exhilarating run it must have been for John and Peter on the way to the tomb of Jesus. Imagine the thoughts going through their heads.

I started running in high school to be with my buddies on the track team. Since then I have run off and on—starting again when my son was two years of age. That first block seemed like miles. Today my wife, Deb, and I run every morning beginning at 5:45 a.m. It is part of our morning routine. Running, jogging, and/or fast walking helps burn extra calories. Keeping those calories under control and in balance requires discipline and determination. Running together also gives us an opportunity to share twenty minutes of uninterrupted conversation. We talk about circumstances and issues that need attention and enjoy each other's company.

I encourage spouses to agree on a regular exercise and prayer time together. If you can't run, walk. If not walking, then ride bikes. Choose something to do together. Call a friend to watch your youngsters or co-op with another couple. Do something active. If you are single, find a friend (or friends) and get moving.

Natural Prescription for Health: If not now—when? If not with him—how about her? What is holding you back? Get up and *get going*!

Personal Thoughts/Goals:

_____

_____

_____

_____

Day 60

Energize Me!

And we desire that each one of you show the same diligence to the full assurance of hope to the end. That you do not become sluggish… (Hebrews 6:11-12).

A common dilemma in our laser-lane society is lack of energy. It is too easy to get a latte, cappuccino, or espresso in the afternoon along with a pastry to pump fuel into the system to get you through until the next fix.

There are many possible reasons for no get-up-and-go. A very common one is that your body does not have enough zinc. (Do not go out and buy zinc now.) Instead, avoid zinc-depleting foods; your body will restore its own reserve of zinc. Zinc is needed to make insulin. Your body uses insulin to put glucose, or fuel, into cells. Zinc levels can be depleted by wheat, soy, and sugar—another reason to limit these items. Vary your grains. Spelt bread is an excellent alternative to wheat.

Low zinc levels may create large facial pores, slow healing time, memory lapses, prostate swelling, and excessive scar or keloid formation. Zinc is balanced with copper. Females with low zinc often have menstrual issues due to the high copper/estrogen connection.

Natural Prescription for Health: Raw pumpkin seeds are a quality source of zinc for everyone. Eat ten or twelve every day.

Personal Thoughts/Goals:

_____

_____

_____

_____

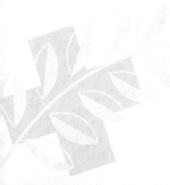

Day 61

Restoring Function

…"Let us rise up and build." Then they set their hands to this good work (Nehemiah 2:18).

"Getting back to the fundamentals" is a common statement used in business, sports, and daily life. The fundamentals are needed to restore function. Optimal health need not elude you. Nehemiah had a purpose that burned with passion—to restore Jerusalem's broken walls and burnt gates. The locals despised Nehemiah's determination and call for action.

Here's a fundamental principle: Clean machines work better. Add measured amounts of pure water to your daily protocol. Your appetite pattern will stabilize, skin integrity will improve, bowels will be consistent, and pain will disappear. Seek food that is organic, fresh, and locally grown. Focus on vegetables, whole grains, and lean meat; avoid wheat and dairy. Do *not* end meals with fruit.

Loosen and relieve tight muscles by using elastic bands to stretch them. Use your bands with outstretched arms in front or behind your trunk. Side bend, twist with your bands, stretch. This basic foundation maneuver promotes flexibility.

Natural Prescription for Health: Aerobically exercise daily for a minimum of thirty minutes—walking or light weight training. Go to sleep by 10:00 p.m. Wake early. Read your Bible daily and meditate on its wisdom; know what you read. Spend time with your family.

Personal Thoughts/Goals:

_____

_____

_____

_____

Day 62

Physically Fit, Kingdom Fit

But Jesus said to him, "No one, having put his hand to the plow, and looking back is fit for the kingdom of God" (Luke 9:62).

What is true in the natural is true in the spiritual. The battle is in the spirit realm (see Eph. 6:10-20). We need to put on the *whole armor of God*—a symbolic and literal event in our lives. Spiritual exercise: Read God's Word, meditate on His Word, pray to the Father; be quiet and listen. Matthew 12:25 says, "...*Every kingdom divided against itself is brought to desolation....*" Move forward in the physical realm.

The first step, which is often the hardest, is to make a decision to become physically and emotionally balanced. Making a positive decision is a move in the right direction—the opposite of working against yourself. Choose to be around people who are proactive self-starters. When you start down the road to optimal health and continue to pursue a healthier you, you will discover how gratified and motivated you become. Do not look back.

Israel looked back to Egypt, and only two people out of millions entered the Promised Land. Joshua and Caleb were hard working proactive optimists. Caleb had the same physical abilities after forty years of wandering, and Joshua replaced Moses as leader. Seek the Lord, follow through and win.

Natural Prescription for Health: Today start your physical and spiritual training regime. Walk and read. Drink water.

Personal Thoughts/Goals:

_____

_____

_____

_____

Day 63

Ducking Diabetes

Weight loss and exercise prevent diabetes more effectively than drugs, says a study of more than three thousand overweight, middle-aged people who had higher-than-normal blood sugar (but not diabetes).[12]

Each person was given either a placebo, Glucophage (a drug used to treat high blood sugar), or sixteen one-on-one sessions to help them lose weight and exercise. After nearly three years, twenty-nine percent of the people in the placebo group had developed diabetes, compared with twenty-two percent of the Glucophage takers. Just fourteen percent of those in the exercise-and-weight-loss group developed diabetes.

The exercisers didn't need to run marathons. Roughly fifty-eight percent of them met the exercise goal (at least two-and-a-half hours a week of moderate aerobic activity, like brisk walking). And thirty-eight percent met the weight-loss goal (they dropped at least seven percent of their body weight by eating a healthy low-calorie, low-fat diet).

Natural Prescription for Health: Get off the couch, office chair, or driver's seat for at least twenty to thirty minutes of walking or other activity every day. Cut calories with a healthy diet that includes lots of fruits and vegetables.

> When I first came to see Dr. Bob, I could not raise my left arm up to my head. It started with neck pain and went down to my shoulder, and my left arm wouldn't function. Since receiving regular adjustments and making a few lifestyle changes, such as eating correctly and regularly exercising, the subluxation has improved and the mobility in my neck is better so that I am now able to turn my head much easier. Also my arm is now functioning normally. The most difficult modification was giving up things containing sugar, as well as yogurt. I was previously on medication for high blood pressure. —Barbara Polen

Personal Thoughts/Goals:

_____

_____

_____

_____

Lunching Naturally

Jesus was aware that the faithful who followed His ministry needed to eat lunch. I would encourage you not to miss any meal. Lunch time is a middle of the day refueling. Your blood sugar does not need a blast of empty fast food or convenience calories. My experience suggests a mixed green salad with protein as a fine midday lunch. Any vegetable raw, steamed, or sautéed, is an option.

As part of the last week of this pattern, you will have the opportunity to record your lunch habits.

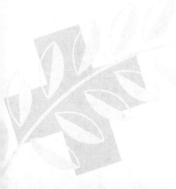

Day 64

"Hold the Pickle"

And the Daughter of Zion…is left like a…booth in a vineyard, like a lodge in a garden of cucumbers, like a besieged city (Isaiah 1:8 AMP).

One of my favorite salad "fixins" is the cucumber. Cucumbers must have been one of the favorites for the Israelites too because it was mentioned, along with garlic, as a food they missed from Egypt. It was also used in biblical times as a refreshing food for feverish patients.

I encourage my patients to use cucumbers as a source of potassium instead of bananas. Bananas have a little more fruit sugar for some individuals to handle, and they tend to constipate. However, if cucumbers (along with green peppers) cause indigestion, it may be time for a liver/gallbladder purge.

Now be aware, cucumbers when "pickled" could be an irritant to your liver. Definitely do not eat a lot of sweet pickles. Cucumbers, Celtic Sea Salt, onions, and organic sour cream make a delightful salad. Onions are also an excellent source of sulfur.

Natural Prescription for Health: Sprinkle dill seed on raw cucumbers for a zesty taste.

Personal Thoughts/Goals:

_____

_____

_____

_____

Day 65

Pass the Mustard

The Kingdom of Heaven is like a mustard seed planted in a field.
It is the smallest of all seeds, but it becomes the largest of garden plants;
it grows into a tree, and birds come and make nests in its branches
(Matthew 13:31-32 NLT).

God has a huge banquet hall waiting for us in Heaven. I am sure mustard will be part of the condiment buffet. Mustard, of which there are many varieties, was spoken about several times in the Bible. The mustard plant or tree has been cultivated worldwide since time began. It even grows wild.

Prior to modern pain relieving medication, mustard, in the form of mustard plaster or mustard paper, was used as a treatment for rheumatism. There are various spices today that have tumeric as one of the ingredients. A very interesting fact: Tumeric, which is sourced from mustard, is a pain reliever. Tumeric prevents the formation of a pain producing tissue-like hormone called Prostaglandin 2.

Natural Prescription for Health: Delete the pain-producing hydrogenated fat in mayonnaise and instead add extra mustard.

Personal Thoughts/Goals:

_____

_____

_____

_____

Day 66

Rustproof Yourself

…where neither moth or rust nor worm consume and destroy… (Matthew 6:20 AMP).

Oxygen is needed for life. We can survive only a brief time without adequate oxygen before our brains will shut down. Likewise, a fire will go out without a source of oxygen.

However, sliced apples will start to discolor when the flesh of the fruit is exposed to the air. This discoloration is a process called oxidation, like rust to car metal. Oxidation is a chemical reaction in which oxygen reacts with another substance, resulting in a chemical transformation. Many of these reactions result in some type of deterioration or spoilage. The purpose of eating antioxidants is to slow down the process of bodily decay.

Blueberries are by far one of the best antioxidants. Fresh greens like spinach also act as a "rustproofer." The more servings of fresh veggies and fruit you eat, the better protected you are against "rust."

Natural Prescription for Health: Fresh or self-frozen blueberries are an excellent year-round source of antioxidants.

Personal Thoughts/Goals:

_____

_____

_____

_____

Day 67

Winning the Pain Game

...Much pain is in every side... (Nahum 2:10).

I have read that up to eighty percent of the US population suffers with some type of pain. Medications have come and gone with high hope and expectation of eliminating some types of pain. Pain caused by an injury, most of the time, heals without any residuals unless it was severe with extreme tissue damage. Insidious, or chronic pain (the annoying type), can literally wear a person out.

Some thoughts: There is a fat, tissue-like hormone called a prostaglandin that can relieve pain. Prostaglandins are part of normal fat metabolism. Yes, fat can relieve your aches and discomfort. I encourage my patients to take one tablespoon of organic flax per one hundred pounds of body weight. This promotes PG3, a pain relieving prostaglandin. Sugar and trans fat inhibit this pain relieving tool.

Natural Prescription for Health: Got milk? Get pain! No milk? Get relief! Exchange cow's milk with almond, rice or coconut milk. The nightshades—tomatoes, white potatoes, green pepper, eggplant, paprika, and peanuts may be an additional little known reason you have pain.

Personal Thoughts/Goals:

_____

_____

_____

_____

Day 68

A Strong Voice

*Your watchman shall lift up their **voices**, with their **voices** they shall sing together...*
(Isaiah 52:8, emphasis added).

I am sure the voice of John the Baptist in the wilderness, with the help of the Holy Spirit, was bold and strong. You might not need a wilderness voice today with the help of technology, but you need to speak without pain or hesitation just the same.

A very common problem I encounter in my practice is a tightening or closing of the vocal region, especially in patients who are stressed. The name of this problem is globus hystericus. I usually see it with patients who have low potassium. Adrenal fatigue (the stress glands located on top of the kidneys) needs minerals including potassium to function at one hundred percent capacity. The vocal cord region can also be congested due to a sulfur deficiency. Sulfur is needed to thin phlegm and drainage and is needed for fat metabolism. Gallbladder distress can create a congested throat region also. Gargle in the shower as this will help strengthen the vocal cords.

Natural Prescription for Health: Grate a sulfur-rich egg on your mixed green lunch salad. Add potassium-rich cucumber slices to your meal.

Personal Thoughts/Goals:

_____

_____

_____

_____

Day 69

Nut Butter

*So their father, Jacob, finally said to them, "If it can't be avoided, then at least do this. Pack your bags with the **best** products of this land. Take them down to the man as gifts— balm, honey, gum, aromatic resin, pistachio nuts, and almonds*
(Genesis 43:11 NLT, emphasis added).

An excellent source of nutrients is from plant-based foods. Plants take in organic minerals from the soil and transfer them into edible, useable building blocks for our use. Think of nuts as seeds for growth. In the Bible, God created seed-bearing plants for our use.

We have been led to believe that peanut butter is an excellent source of protein and that it is good for you. First, peanuts are not nuts. They are legumes and can actually be considered a nightshade (plants with poisonous juice). Peanuts have a certain little-known toxin as a part of their makeup called aflatoxin. I have seen from experience that peanuts can cause an issue with yeast. Peanut butter, eaten straight, or on sandwiches can be the main reason for your chronic dripping nose. One patient's fifty-year-old sinus problem cleared up just by eliminating peanut butter from his diet.

Natural Prescription for Health: Do you suffer from chronic sinus pain? Try eating almond or cashew butter.

Personal Thoughts/Goals:

_____

_____

_____

_____

Day 70

Good for the Heart

People who eat beans, almond butter, and other legumes at least four times a week have a twenty-one percent lower risk of heart disease than those who eat legumes less than once a week, says a nineteen-year study of nearly ten thousand people.[13]

The researchers couldn't say, though, why bean-eaters have healthier hearts. Among the possible reasons: beans have soluble fiber, which lowers cholesterol, and folate, which can lower blood levels of homocysteine, an amino acid that promotes heart disease.

Natural Prescription for Health: Eat more beans. Think of them not as beans, but as chick pea curry, split pea soup, rice and lentils, burritos, hummus, and pasta e fagioli.

> I came to see Dr. Bob because I was suffering with sinus infections. I would get a bad infection three to four times a month, and a sinus specialist recommended that I have surgery. I asked Dr. Bob if he could help me, and after running some tests and looking at my x-rays, he said that he could. Before coming to see Dr. Bob, I was on and off twelve to thirteen medicines for my sinuses without much relief. Since following Dr.'s recommendations, I haven't had a sinus infection. My health has improved a lot. I have more energy since I am not sick all the time. I would like to thank God for giving Dr. Bob the knowledge he has about natural healthcare. —Paula Hall

Personal Thoughts/Goals:

_____

_____

_____

_____

Day 71

Detoxification

Cleanse me with hyssop and I shall be clean; wash me, and I shall be whiter than snow
(Psalm 51:7).

We live in a very toxic environment. I focus a large percent of my patient contact time on detoxification. Detoxifying starts by stopping. You need to stop consuming processed food, human-made oils, sugar, and artificial colors. You might be thinking, "Dr. Bob, everything I eat is processed and colored." My response: eat food without labels. You find them in the produce department, not in the prepared food department—ninety percent of the aisle space in our grocery stores.

We dump nearly one hundred billion pounds of toxic material in our fifty-five thousand garbage dump sites in the US. The EPA states that forty percent of our fresh water is unfit for use, much less drinking. We are exposed to toxins through lawn applications, oven cleaners, home pesticides, paint cleaners, vehicle exhaust, the lawn trash, and so forth. Even in a relatively clean environment, our cells accumulate waste products as a part of normal living.

Modern herbalists consider hyssop to be one of more outstanding herbs for detoxification of the colon. It was important in Abraham's time and is even more important today.

Natural Prescription for Health: Add raw, grated organic beets to your salad to help your liver get cleansed.

Personal Thoughts/Goals:

_____

_____

_____

_____

Day 72

Food for Thought

So He humbled you, allowed you to hunger, and fed you with manna which you did not know nor did your fathers know, that He might make you know that man shall not live by bread alone; but man lives by every word that proceeds from the mouth of the Lord (Deuteronomy 8:3).

What should you eat to think clearly? How can you have the mind of Christ? What did Jesus feed on? The Word, the Bread of Life.

The brain is made of fat. Eating the right fat or nutrients to make brain fat promotes brain health. Do you know your brain needs phosphorous lipids? A great source of brain food is Omega 3 fats found in marine life and selected green plants. Your brain also needs neurotransmitters. I encourage my patients to eat protein. Your body will utilize vitamin B6 to help convert protein to neurotransmitters. Vitamin B6 is commonly deficient in individuals who use birth control pills.

You could have your liver enzymes checked. Low liver enzymes may be a result of insufficient B6. Breads with whole grains and olive oil or flax oil substituted for butter is also a great way to feed the brain. Do not eat margarine.

Natural Prescription for Health: Add chicken, turkey, or lamb to your mixed green salad lunch.

Personal Thoughts/Goals:

_____

_____

_____

_____

Day 73

What About Cheese?

And carry these ten cheeses to the captain of their thousand, and see how your brothers fare, and bring back news of them (1 Samuel 17:18).

Jesse, David's very smart dad, was aware of the value of cheese as a gift. He incorporated the law of reciprocity for the favor and safety of his sons by blessing their commander with ten wheels of cheese, while engaging Goliath. Goat's milk, it has been suggested, is similar to human milk. (It sure doesn't smell or taste appetizing.) Goat cheese was a common staple of the biblical diet. The process of fermentation and enzyme action was not altered by heat or chemicals like it is today.

Cheese is a logical way to incorporate dairy into your life. However, in my experience, most patients can only tolerate a small amount of cheese before they notice left neck pain, general body pain, skin eruptions, or other toxic overload symptoms including sinusitis. Focus on raw, organic cheese without additives. This quality can be located in most grocery stores today. Do not eat human-made cheese in a can, box, or with colors and additives. Be sensitive to body symptoms with the addition of cheese in your diet.

Natural Prescription for Health: Chevre goat cheese with fresh basil, olive oil, and thin sliced tomatoes is a refreshing treat.

Personal Thoughts/Goals:

_____

_____

_____

_____

Day 74

Blind as a Bat

*And the men who journeyed with him stood speechless, hearing
a voice but seeing no one* (Acts 9:7).

Bats generally fly at night. They see with vibrations or sonar. Bats emit a source of energy and effectively navigate by analyzing patterns. We can see easily during the day with sunlight, but struggle to see without light at night. The dark circle or pupil in the center of the eye responds to the amount of light in the environment.

Your eyesight is affected by the nutrients you eat. Eyes require an excellent blood supply and vitamin A. Challenges of night vision impairment can improve by eating a quality source of organic carrots. Fresh, raw carrots are best. Floaters in your eyes diminish with vitamin A and liver cleansing. The liver uses and stores vitamin A. When the liver is short on vitamin A, it "borrows" it from the eyes. You can juice carrots, drinking eight ounces at one time. Always drink it fresh.

Natural Prescription for Health: A need for sunglasses suggests a need for potassium-rich cucumbers.

Personal Thoughts/Goals:

_____

_____

_____

_____

Day 75

Give Us Our Daily Bread

Give us this day our daily bread (Matthew 6:11).

In the Lord's Prayer, our Heavenly Father wanted to make sure we had our daily bread, physically from grain and spiritually from His Word, the Bread of Life. Let's talk about bread.

I have found from experience that all wheat sources, yes whole wheat—albino white wheat, styrofoam-fake white wheat—may be a problem for some people. I have seen chronic allergies eliminated by ceasing to eat wheat products. Test yourself. Go without wheat for one month. The protein in wheat, called gluten, can create an "alarm attack" by the body. Headaches, body pain, sinusitis, digestive distress, and even tremors can be a reaction to wheat. I have seen relief in people within days, especially if they daily ate wheat bagels, toast, sandwiches, hoagies, pizza, and so forth.

A possible substitute can be spelt grain bread. Spelt does not appear to create distress in most patients. Rotate your grains: brown rice, almond meal, amaranth, and gluten-free oat flour. Always put some type of oil on your bread, such as olive or flax. It appears that wheat sensitivities may be associated with a B6 and "good" oil deficiency.

Natural Prescription for Health: Substitute spelt bread for wheat bread. Limit your bread consumption.

Personal Thoughts/Goals:

_____

_____

_____

_____

Day 76

Curds From Cattle

Did you not pour me out like milk, and curdle me like cheese… (Job 10:10).

Curds have been described as cheese and butter in the Bible. I normally advise my patients to avoid commercially-made cottage cheese. However, there are some who would suggest that the protein in the curds along with flax oil assist the body in controlling cancer. I have no experience in this thought. I have seen, from decades of experience, though, that dairy items such as milk, cottage cheese, and ice cream can be the primary cause of pain.

You need to be a label reader and study the ingredients in any dairy product you ingest. Always be mindful of sugar, high fructose corn syrup, and evaporated cane juice or crystals. Look for any mention of artificial colors. Sweeteners and colors cause additional stress on the lymph, liver, and digestive systems.

If you have little or no pain, sinus, digestive, or skin issues and want to add some cheese to a sandwich, casserole, or special meal, by all means do it. My concern for you is that dairy can be the one item with which the media has bombarded you, suggesting that it is necessary for your existence. Let me assure you that I have thousands of patients from all ages who thrive without milk. Butter is better than margarine and is considered by Udo Erasamus, author of *Fats That Heal—Fats that Kill,* to be a neutral food, not adding or taking away from your optimal health, when studied in a pros and cons list.

Natural Prescription for Health: Conventionally-raised cattle are medicated with antibiotics, growth hormones, and steroids. Focus on organic dairy items.

Personal Thoughts/Goals:

_____

_____

_____

_____

Day 77

Salad Savvy

Will you walk away from the table with fewer calories if you start your meal with a salad? It depends on the salad.

Researchers had forty-two women eat as much pasta as they wanted for lunch, with or without one of several salads before the pasta. The women ate twelve percent fewer calories when they were given a large salad (three cups) with low calorie density (veggies plus fat-free dressing and light cheese) than when they ate pasta alone.

Even after a small (one-and-a-half cup) salad, they ate seven percent fewer calories than when they were offered pasta alone.

However, when the women ate either a large or small *calorie-dense* salad (with regular dressing and cheese), they ended up consuming *more* calories than when they ate only pasta.[14]

Natural Prescription for Health: Start dinner with a salad that is mostly vegetables. If you aren't a fan of fat-free dressing, try organic reduced-fat (as little as possible) and skip the cheese, croutons, Chinese noodles, and other calorie-dense salad trimmings.

> I had been suffering with asthma, allergies, and colds. I had an inhaler that I carried everywhere along with medications. The information and care provided by Dr. DeMaria has improved my life. My asthma and allergies are gone, and I don't get sick any more. Following Dr. Bob's advice, I cut sugar and dairy out of my diet. Every time I went back to my old eating habits, my asthma and allergies came back. —Jason Lance

Personal Thoughts/Goals:

_____

_____

_____

_____

Day 78

Accelerated Healing

He was wounded for our transgressions, He was bruised for our guilt and iniquities...
(Isaiah 53:5 AMP).

Jesus was bruised for our iniquity. We have been healed by the stripes Jesus took for us. We have everlasting life because of His obedience. Patients who heal slowly, in the natural, often have a zinc deficiency. Slow healers with excess scarring normally have low zinc and high copper. Bruising easily and without cause could be due to aspirin, blood thinners, and salmon oil use.

Seniors with poor oxygenation to tissues can have bruising on the lower forearms. The unexplained, for-no-reason bruises are always a concern. Blood cells generally circulate about 120 days. Healing will take time. Blood loss from a heavy menstrual flow or through the rectum needs to be evaluated. I encourage my patients to eat a mixed green salad for lunch. Greens are an excellent source of chlorophyll, which promotes vitamin K utilization. Lack of vitamin C can also result in bruising. The blood system is the oxygen carrying health promoting system. Life begets life.

Natural Prescription for Health: Bruising easily and without cause? I would discuss a prothrombin time test evaluation with your healthcare provider. Eat more greens and raw bell peppers.

Personal Thoughts/Goals:

_____

_____

_____

Lunch Journal:

_____

_____

_____

Day 79

Prevent Pestilence

*Nor the pestilence that walks in darkness, nor of the destruction
that lays waste at noonday (Psalm 91:6).*

Pestilence can be any event or condition, internal or external, that interferes with your ability to thrive as God intended. A modern-day pestilence, unlike locusts or grasshoppers in biblical times, which were seasonal or short-lived, is cancer. I applaud the progress that has been achieved so far, but is irradiating and injecting chemicals into a body with a stressed immune system the logical approach?

We have helped many with body breakdown. You must change the lifestyle you had that allowed the cancer cells to proliferate. Clean machines work the best. Do you have a family history of cancer? Change the recipe box; avoid foods that are fried. Obesity creates stress on an already congested liver and is common in cancer patients. Drink water. Eat fresh, organic produce. Stop smoking and avoid beverages that need to be processed by the liver—such as alcohol and diet soda.

Natural Prescription for Health: Clean livers are healthy livers. Grate raw beets onto your salad—today!

Personal Thoughts/Goals:

_____

_____

_____

_____

Lunch Journal:

_____

_____

_____

_____

Day 80

Sandwiches

Where could we get enough bread in the wilderness to fill such a great multitude?
(Matthew 15:33).

A common staple in the American diet is a sandwich. There are deli sandwiches, hoagies, footlongs, hot dogs, quarter pounders, half pounders, and so forth. The ingredients in a typical lunch meal appear healthy enough; however, deli meats are generally loaded with salty preservatives and coloring.

Are you thirsty after a meal? Your body is attempting to dilute the poison you just consumed. The mayo is made of difficult-to-process trans fat, sugar-loaded catsup, and relish. What is the source of the "white" enriched bread? Combining protein (meat requiring acid to digest) along with carbohydrates (bread requiring alkalinity) confuses the system. I have noticed that patients in my practice with blood type A tend to have more challenges digesting a sandwich versus those with blood type O. Loading up veggies between whole-grain bread is a safe option. Do you want deli meat? Buy an organic variety that does not contain hormones or preservatives. Roll up a slice with your favorite veggies or lettuce, and chew it thoroughly. Your stomach will thank you.

Natural Prescription for Health: Nut butter sandwiches are a digestive safe alternative to meat-based favorites.

Personal Thoughts/Goals:

_____

_____

_____

Lunch Journal:

_____

_____

_____

_____

Day 81

Peppermint Leaves

Woe to you scribes and Pharisees, pretenders (hypocrites)! For you give a tenth of your mint and dill and cummin, and have neglected and omitted the weightier...matters of the Law (Matthew 23:23 AMP).

There must have been some value to mint in the New Testament since Jesus made mention of it in regard to the Pharisees paying a tithe on it. The exact variety is not mentioned, but all mints are very aromatic.

I personally enjoy herbal peppermint tea. We have it growing in direct sunlight in our front yard. It is a perennial plant that shows up annually. The flavor is very stimulating to the palate—it will put a little spring in your step. The essential oil obtained from mint leaves contains menthol, which is used as a cooling remedy. It is also great to add the leaves to water and lemon. The refreshing mint zest can also be used as a replacement for caffeinated tea or soda. Add the mint leaves as a garnish when serving leg of lamb. The leaves are edible—your mouth will come alive with one bite.

Natural Prescription for Health: Add peppermint leaves to your favorite herbal tea.

Personal Thoughts/Goals:

_____

_____

_____

_____

Lunch Journal:

_____

_____

_____

_____

Day 82

Skip the Milk

*For everyone who partakes **only of milk** is unskilled in the word of righteousness, for he is a babe. But solid food belongs to those who are of full age, that is, those who by reason of use have their senses exercised to discern both good and evil* (Hebrews 5:13, emphasis added).

From my experience, a majority of the chronic "no known causes" of body pain and breakdown are sugar, human-made fat, and milk. Healthier human beings were raised on breast milk and whole food. Patients who were raised on formula and cow-based dairy products tend to have more ear infections, skin problems, asthma, bowel issues, and joint pain.

Substances derived from cow's milk are more difficult to digest. Protein in milk can create chronic allergies. Cow's milk has more calcium for cow bones and less phospholipids for brains. The million dollar question: Where do cows get their calcium? Ice cream, cottage cheese, yogurt, or milk? No! They eat hay, grass, and alfalfa. Now I don't want you to go out and graze in the field, but eating living food does make sense.

Seriously, do you crave cow's milk? Consume sesame seeds for calcium; flax oil for fat, chicken and turkey for protein. These three items resolve most cow milk desires.

Natural Prescription for Health: Try unsweetened coconut milk or rice milk novelties as an alternative to dairy-sourced ice cream.

Personal Thoughts/Goals:

_____

_____

_____

Lunch Journal:

_____

_____

_____

Day 83

Dr. Bob's Lunch

*And Jesus took the loaves, and when He had given thanks He distributed
them to the disciples, and the disciples to those sitting down;
and likewise the fish, as much as they wanted (John 6:11).*

What does the manual say? Premium, plus, or regular fuel? The grade, quality, and octane (or fire power) of the fuel affects the peak performance of acceleration. Do you putter after lunch? Lack of quality B vitamins can cause drowsiness. Consuming a carbohydrate meal without protein for lunch creates a desire for sweets for your midday fueling around 3:00 p.m. Protein is like a slow burning log keeping the machine working steady as she goes.

Avoid heavy starchy meals such as pasta, rice, and/or potatoes for lunch. Focus on steamed veggies and protein—chicken, turkey, tuna, beef, without bread. Those pieces of bread add up in calories. Limit beverages to a sip or two of water—and say no to soda. Use fresh cucumbers, bell peppers, or tomatoes to provide the liquid to digest food so you will be able minimize water while chewing and swallowing. Water dilutes your weakened stomach acid. Drink water one-half hour before or after meals. Do not get in the habit of drinking alcohol at lunch time. Do not eat fruit at the end of the meal.

I eat a mixed green (no iceberg) salad that includes: radishes, tomatoes, cucumbers, beets, sesame and sunflower seeds, cauliflower, broccoli, cabbage, carrots and parsley, chives or basil. I use flax oil and beet juice for my dressing. Enjoy!

Natural Prescription for Health: Mixed greens with protein is the midday fuel for champions.

Personal Thoughts/Goals:

_____

_____

Lunch Journal:

_____

_____

Day 84

Whole Grains and Diabetes

Why ask for that sandwich on whole wheat bread? People who eat whole grains have a lower risk of diabetes, say researchers at the University of Minnesota and elsewhere.

Lawrence Kushi and colleagues gave diet questionnaires to nearly thirty-six thousand healthy Iowa women aged fifty-five to sixty-nine when the study began in 1986. After six years, 1,141 of the women had been diagnosed with diabetes.

Those who consumed the most whole grains (average: three servings a day) had a twenty-one percent lower risk of diabetes than those who consumed the least (average: once a week). Those who consumed the most fiber (average: ten grams a day) from breads, cereals, and other grains had a twenty-nine percent lower risk than those who consumed the least (average: three grams a day). (Fruit and vegetable fiber wasn't linked to diabetes.) And those who consumed the most magnesium, a mineral found in whole grains, had a twenty-four percent lower risk than those who consumed the least.

"Being overweight is clearly an overwhelming risk factor for the development of diabetes, and physical activity is important, too," says Kushi, who is now at Columbia University. "But there is growing evidence that whole grains also play a role. It's just hard to know whether it's their fiber, magnesium, or something else that matters."[15]

> Before making Dr. Bob's suggested lifestyle changes, I had been suffering with chronic ear irritations as well as hip pain for twenty-five years on and off. I was on medication for cholesterol and blood pressure, and I was on Wellbutrin for nerves. I have modified my food intake. I now eat more natural foods and drink lots of water. Giving up treats with sugar has been difficult. However, I no longer take medications for cholesterol and blood pressure. My ear infections are a thing of the past. The aura in Dr. Bob's office is like a warm hug! It makes me feel really "cared about." Like a loving family! —Judy Kuenzel

Personal Thoughts/Goals:

_____

_____

Lunch Journal:

_____

_____

Self-Assessment
Lunch Debriefing

Using the information you wrote in your Lunch Journals, answer the following questions and mark your score as directed. Your goal is a score of five.

_____ Did you eat lunch each day? Add one.

_____ Did you focus on mixed greens (with olive or flax oil), lightly steamed veggies with animal or plant protein? Add one.

_____ Did you eat a fast food meal with trans fat or partially hydrogenated oil? Subtract one.

_____ What beverage did you have? Water, water with lemon, herbal tea, (4 ounces only?) No change.

_____ Did you drink coffee (decaf or regular), soda, eight ounces or more of water, a dairy product, caffeine tea? Subtract one.

_____ Did you have a refined grain bread product, hoagie, wheat bun, bread, pasta, or pastry? Subtract one.

_____ Did you have a sprouted grain, spelt, millet, rice flour, or other whole grain alone or with a nut or plant protein? Add one.

_____ Did you have a dessert? Subtract one.

_____ Did you end your meal with fruit? Subtract one.

_____ Did you eat in your vehicle? Subtract one.

_____ Did you use peanut butter? Subtract one. Any other nut butter, add one.

_____ Did you have animal protein and starch together? Subtract one.

_____ Did you use olive or flax oil? Add one.

_____ Did you eat your own prepared food? Fresh or left over? Add one.

_____ Did you consume alcohol? Subtract one.

_____ Total score

Dr. Bob's lunch comment: Your goal is to eat a light meal in the midday. Adding fruit or dessert on a layer of protein and starches creates the potential for digestive distress.

Gluten may be a stealth cause of a variety of health challenges, including headaches, pain, dark circles under your eyes, digestive distress, and many more. Gluten is a protein found in these commonly used grains: wheat, rye, oats, and barley. I would suggest, if you have chronic health challenges and have been journaling your meals and notice the above mentioned foods, you may consider going gluten-free for a month. Then have a gluten festival—eating bread, pasta, and pizza, and see if the symptoms that went away come back. Barley is often used as a base ingredient for caramel coloring used in sodas and items desiring a "natural" brown color.

If going gluten-free does not give you pain relief or if other chronic health challenges continue to linger, you may then want to consider going on a nightshade–free lifestyle for four to six weeks: no tomatoes, white potatoes, green peppers, hot peppers, eggplant, peanuts, or paprika. This regime may seem a bit demanding, but I have learned from experience that pain has everything to do with what you are putting in and on your body.

Meal Prep

Meal preparation along with understanding food combinations is essential. What you eat, when you eat, and with whom you eat has an influence on the final product that enters the cell. I generally see optimal health in patients who do not eat their meals with a dessert. Animal protein mixes best with non-starch food like broccoli, cabbage, beans, and mixed greens. Avoid pastas, grain, and potatoes with animal protein. It's always more beneficial to eat fruit alone, without combining it with other food.

Do you have digestive distress? This new pattern will go far in helping to minimize discomfort. You will notice improvement, I promise!

Food Combination Charts

Foods properly combined streamline digestion, promote weight loss, and energize and strengthen your entire body.

Fruit

Eat fruit by itself on an empty stomach. Let twenty to thirty minutes elapse after eating fruit before eating other foods.

Acid Fruit

Blackberries	Plums (Sour)
Grapefruit	Pomegranate
Kumquat	Raspberries
Lemon	Strawberries
Lime	Tangerines
Orange	Tangelos
Pineapple	

Sub-Acid Fruit

Apple	Kiwi
Apricot	Loquat
Blueberries	Nectarine
Cherimoya	Papaya
Cherries	Peach
Fresh Fig	Pear
Grapes	Plums (Sweet)
Huckleberries	

Sweet Fruit

Bananas
Dates
Dried Fruit
Grapes (Thompson & Muscat)
Persimmon
Raisins

Melon

Cantaloupe	Honeydew
Casaba	Musk
Christmas	Sharlyn
Persian Melon	Watermelon
Crenshaw	

Note: Ideally Sweet Fruits should be eaten after other fruits

Note: Ideally Melon should be eaten alone or before other fruits

Note: Three hours should elapse after eating cooked foods before eating fruit again.

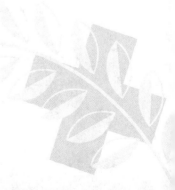

Protein and Starches

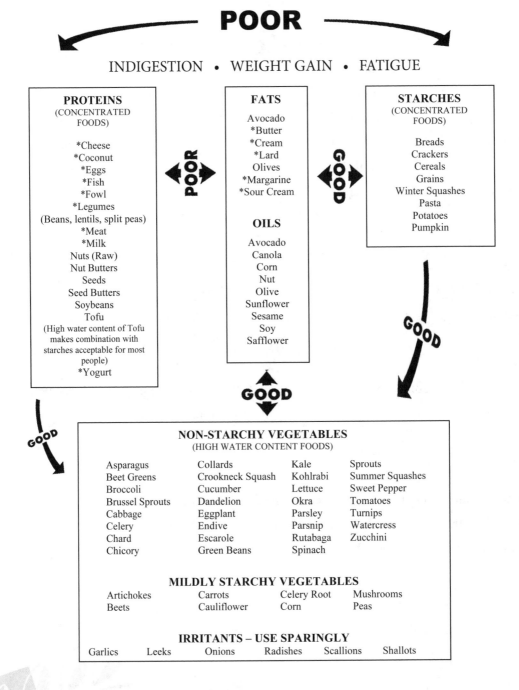

POOR

INDIGESTION • WEIGHT GAIN • FATIGUE

PROTEINS
(CONCENTRATED FOODS)

*Cheese
*Coconut
*Eggs
*Fish
*Fowl
*Legumes
(Beans, lentils, split peas)
*Meat
*Milk
Nuts (Raw)
Nut Butters
Seeds
Seed Butters
Soybeans
Tofu
(High water content of Tofu makes combination with starches acceptable for most people)
*Yogurt

FATS
Avocado
*Butter
*Cream
*Lard
Olives
*Margarine
*Sour Cream

OILS
Avocado
Canola
Corn
Nut
Olive
Sunflower
Sesame
Soy
Safflower

STARCHES
(CONCENTRATED FOODS)

Breads
Crackers
Cereals
Grains
Winter Squashes
Pasta
Potatoes
Pumpkin

POOR **GOOD** **GOOD** **GOOD**

NON-STARCHY VEGETABLES
(HIGH WATER CONTENT FOODS)

Asparagus	Collards	Kale	Sprouts
Beet Greens	Crookneck Squash	Kohlrabi	Summer Squashes
Broccoli	Cucumber	Lettuce	Sweet Pepper
Brussel Sprouts	Dandelion	Okra	Tomatoes
Cabbage	Eggplant	Parsley	Turnips
Celery	Endive	Parsnip	Watercress
Chard	Escarole	Rutabaga	Zucchini
Chicory	Green Beans	Spinach	

MILDLY STARCHY VEGETABLES

Artichokes	Carrots	Celery Root	Mushrooms
Beets	Cauliflower	Corn	Peas

IRRITANTS – USE SPARINGLY

Garlics   Leeks   Onions   Radishes   Scallions   Shallots

Note: Proteins and starches eaten together tend to spoil in the stomach.

Note: Eat *proteins* as a main course with vegetables and/or salad.

Note: Eat *starches* as a main course with vegetables and/or salad.

Day 85

Food Combinations

Then he [Noah] *drank of the wine and was drunk, and became uncovered in his tent*
(Genesis 9:21).

Eating food without thought of consequences results in conditions that are often difficult to correct. Most patients I have observed from diet journal analysis eat a limited variety of foods. Food rotation, which is adding and deleting food groups, consistently promotes health. Habits are challenging to change. Breakfast cereals, sandwiches, dining out for dinner, or eating prepared, purchased food is the norm. Forty-seven percent of the American food budget is spent on meals consumed out of the home.

I encourage patients to eat fruit alone and in the morning, followed by nuts. The nuts limit insulin release. I strongly suggest eliminating fruits after a meal. Eating fruit after a meal results in slowed or delayed digestion and fermentation. Fermentation of undigested food in a warm, dark environment (your stomach) produces poison gases, foul-smelling stools, and if the combination is right, even alcohol. Some people appear to be in a fog or unfocused—they may be in a subclinical alcohol stupor. I have seen elevated liver enzymes in patients who combine fruits with meals and do not even drink alcohol. Check your own food journal. What do you see?

Natural Prescription for Health: Eat fruit alone in the morning.

Personal Thoughts/Goals:

_____

_____

_____

_____

Day 86

You Are What You Eat, Digest, Absorb

*…The priest's servant would come with a three-pronged fleshhook in his hand while the meat was **boiling** (1 Samuel 2:13, emphasis added).*

Digestive distress prevents your body from gathering the nutrients you need to have optimal health. Correct food choices are critical. Avoid processed, devitalized food.

Cooking methods affect the quality of the end product. Boiling draws the minerals and vitamins out of the fiber into the water and down the drain. Raw, lightly steamed, or blanched veggies go a long way in providing your digestive system enzymes for assimilation. Taking time to slowly chew bathes food, especially starch food, with enzymes needed for digestion. Minimize water while chewing and swallowing. Water dilutes your weakened stomach acid. Drink water one-half hour before or after meals. Incidentally, water is absorbed in the large intestine.

Fiber food such as broccoli, cabbage, beans, and apples are necessary to keep your colon moving. Digestion starts in the mouth and ends in the colon.

Natural Prescription for Health: Steam your vegetables versus boiling them.

Personal Thoughts/Goals:

_____

_____

_____

_____

Day 87

You Are the Salt of the Earth

You are the salt of the earth, but if salt has lost its taste…how can its saltness be restored (Matthew 5:13 AMP).

Salt is one of those minerals that is misunderstood. Salt at one point in time was used as a source of payment—like money. People were paid in salt.

Today, people shy away from salt because they have been told that salt will raise their blood pressure. I do not want you to throw your shaker out, and I do not want you to binge on salt; however, only five percent of blood pressure issues are connected to salt. I encourage my patients to use a salt called Celtic Sea Salt. It is sourced from France and has not been whitened, colored, or altered in any way. I also recommend that patients shy away from sodium-chloride or any salt that has additives.

Sodium is a mineral. Your body needs minerals. Craving salt is often a sign of weak adrenal function. Adrenal glands make hormones in the body including cortisone. You need real, quality salt!

Natural Prescription for Health: Liberally use Celtic Sea Salt®. Find this product in most health food stores.

Personal Thoughts/Goals:

_____

_____

_____

_____

Day 88

Shoulder Pain

*The God of this people Israel chose our fathers and exalted the people when they dwelt as strangers in the land of Egypt, and with an **uplifted arm** He brought them out of it* (Acts 13:17, emphasis added).

God had use of all His limbs. Raising arms and shoulders is a sign of strength. Aaron supported Moses' arms during a fatigued state, guaranteeing victory (see Exod. 17:12).

Can you raise your arms above your head without pain? There is a common condition that affects the tissues around the muscles and bones of the shoulder called bursitis. A bursae is a sac that separates layers of tissue protecting them from being irritated. Think of it as a liquid cushion. In my experience I have seen more often in females around thirty-five to forty years old (any age or gender can be effected) pain below the shoulder tip, in the mid-arm. The condition is bursitis.

Bursitis is often associated with an alkaline saliva pH (purple-color test paper). Citrus consumption including oranges, grapefruits, and tangerines or juice may be the cause of the higher pH. B6 supplementation along with organic apple cider vinegar may be needed for a season.

Natural Prescription for Health: Do not drink fluids with your meals. This tends to raise saliva pH.

Personal Thoughts/Goals:

_____

_____

_____

_____

Day 89

Lemon Zest

And you shall take for yourselves on the first day the fruit of beautiful trees
(Leviticus 23:40 NKJV, emphasis added).

According to rabbis, the fruit of "goodly trees" means lemons.

I thoroughly enjoy watching the Food Channel on TV or, better yet, going to a culinary class. I recently learned about zest at one class. Purchase organic lemons and wash them thoroughly. You need a grater with small sharp surfaces for cutting. Grate some lemon skin or peel and add it to your favorite marinade for your gas grill or broiler. I generally use Paul Newman's Oil and Vinegar, which doesn't contain sugar. Spread the mixture on chicken—boy, does it add some pizzazz!

Another suggestion is to cut a lemon into fourths. Take one wedge and squeeze it into hot water. Sip on the water and eat the lemon. This is great for a morning beverage, cleansing the liver and kidneys. Kidney stones cause intense pain. I've witnessed that drinking one lemon wedge in eight ounces of hot water every fifteen minutes can either minimize the pain or cause the stones to pass naturally.

A simple snoring remedy is to drink hot water with a wedge of lemon juice added and then eat the lemon right before bed. Try it! A caution: If my patients have fibromyalgia, I encourage them to minimize citrus and be aware of any changes while ingesting lemons.

Natural Prescription for Health: Try a cup of water with a fresh lemon wedge, stevia (an herb to sweeten), and mint leaves as a beverage.

Personal Thoughts/Goals:

_____

_____

_____

_____

Day 90

Cooking Tips

*If your grain offering is prepared on a griddle, it is to be made
of fine flour mixed with oil, and without yeast* (Leviticus 2:5 NIV).

So what type of pots and pans do you use to cook? We use stainless steel Cuisinart®
cookware. We also bake frequently in our oven using baking bags, which prevent loss
of nutrients and reduce cooking time. I bake beets every week, and I also consistently bake
chicken and turkey in the oven. As a side note, in my experience, I have not noticed an
elevation in hair analysis aluminum levels in individuals who use aluminum cookware.

The poorest nutritional method of cooking food is boiling. The quality of water is
significant, and the length of time the item is heated affects the content and value of
nutrients left. Boiling draws the nutrient into the water and then the water (and nutrient)
is poured down the drain. Baked sweet potatoes and yams are more nutritious than
boiled and mashed. The least amount of heat applied to your meal, the more usable
nutrients are available for cell restoration.

You can spray olive, high oleic safflower, or sunflower oils from a manual pump
sprayer instead of commercially produced hydrogenated "low cholesterol" products.
Butter can also be used as a source of frying fat.

Natural Prescription for Health: Heat destroys nutrients. Always have raw veggies
with a meal providing enzymes that give your pancreas a breather.

Personal Thoughts/Goals:

_____

_____

_____

_____

Day 91

Never Too Late

Want to stick around to see your great-grandchildren? In a study of more than 2,300 people in eleven European countries, those who ate a healthy Mediterranean diet, exercised, didn't smoke, and drank alcohol moderately were more likely to live into their eighties and beyond. The researchers gave the highest diet scores to people who ate less meat, dairy, and saturated fat and more fruits, vegetables, beans, fish, grains, nuts, and unsaturated fats. People with the highest scores had a twenty-three percent lower risk of dying during the ten-year study.

Not smoking and staying physically active each cut the risk about thirty-five percent. People who drank alcohol moderately had a twenty-two percent lower risk. And the folks who scored high on all four measures were sixty-five percent less likely to die of any cause, including heart disease and cancer.[16]

Natural Prescription for Health: All of the above. Just don't equate a Mediterranean diet with pizza or lasagna. And don't use the study as an excuse to start drinking.

I had a lot of lower back pain, depression, and excessive weight. My biggest health problem was an addiction to narcotic pain medication. I was taking six different medications. Following Dr. DeMaria's recommendations, I changed my eating habits and began regular exercise. I also take time for prayer and reading, which has helped break my addiction. I still struggle with my diet, but my husband and I are always learning and trying new things to eat. I am now down to only two of my medications. Words will never express how Dr. Bob and Debbie have invested in our health. Our change has been like night and day; we are new people. I feel fifteen years younger! I just want to say "thank you" for your ministry. You have balanced physically, mentally, and spiritually. Dr. Bob, you inspire my mind, body, and soul! —Debra Arabian

Personal Thoughts/Goals:

_____

_____

_____

_____

Day 92

The New Recipe Box

Do not remember the former things, nor consider the things of old [unhealthy recipes].
Behold, I will do a new thing... (Isaiah 43:18-19).

You cannot go forward looking in the rear view mirror. Are you satisfied with your current level of health? What can you do to minimize pain, sleep better, lose weight, and have more energy? What is the state of your family's health? Mom, Dad, Grandma, Grandpa, aunts, uncles, sisters, brothers?

Health states are not all necessarily genetically passed on. Are you thumbing through the same "family recipes"? I have treated five generations in families. The members who choose high amounts of carbohydrates from grains, pastas, and nutrient-dense, low-fiber foods appear to be heavier and more sickly and have more health issues than members from the same family who focus on eating low grains and pastas and include more greens and proteins. You are what you eat.

Ask happy, healthy-looking people what they eat. Copy their recipes.

Natural Prescription for Health: Change what's in your recipe box if your traditional family meals perpetuate poor health. Heavy, rich ethnic foods promote liver stress.

Personal Thoughts/Goals:

_____

_____

_____

_____

Day 93

Herbs Are a Blessing

For the earth which drinks in the rain that often comes upon it, and bears **herbs** *useful for those by whom it is cultivated receives blessing from God* (Hebrews 6:7, emphasis added).

Our Heavenly Father has provided food and drink from the beginning. Herbs have been a part of that plan since Genesis. There are many classifications of herbs. Herbs have been used to tone, excite, and relax the body and mind.

I have several planting boxes on my deck at home where I grow herbs. In the springtime, shop at a greenhouse nursery or health food store for organic herbs plants or seeds. This is when you will have the best selection.

Parsley has many varieties. It is an excellent kidney purifier. I suggest, especially with individuals with kidney stress, to eat parsley on their mixed green salads or steep it in hot water and drink it as a tea. Chives add the essence of onion. They are great in scrambled eggs, salads, macaroni, and potato dishes. Dill adds an exciting zest to food. Sage and rosemary are very bold—only use a pinch. Thyme and oregano are awesome in tomato sauce. We snip basil with kitchen sheers. It's tasty with thin tomato slices and olive oil.

Natural Prescription for Health: Make it a priority to buy, plant, and water your three favorite herbs. Use them!

Personal Thoughts/Goals:

_____

_____

_____

_____

Day 94

Chicken Soup for the Soul

As fire burns brushwood, as fire causes water to boil… (Isaiah 64:2).

My friend Mark Victor Hansen, co-author of the *Chicken Soup* book series, reaffirmed the healing virtue of food. The chicken soup I want to discuss is not from a can, foil pack, recycled container, or bottle.

Real chicken soup starts with fresh organic chicken, especially thighs and legs. There are natural ingredients in animal protein that stimulate the immune system. Start with quality water, filtered with reverse osmosis. Boil the chicken and a whole onion until tender. The only time you want to boil anything is when making soups or sauces because boiling, then draining, eliminates essential nutrients. A lid is useful to keep everything in the pot. Let the chicken cool; debone all the meat and set it aside. Cut up the onion along with celery and carrots and add to the stock (water flavored by the cooked chicken). Simmer—I normally let it simmer 30 to 40 minutes. Add chicken meat, fresh parsley, and Celtic Sea Salt. Let the mixture slowly cook for at least an hour, or until your salivating from the awesome aroma gets the best of you. Prepare brown rice. When all the flavors are blended, ladle out some fresh, soul-refreshing and body-nourishing soup and rice. Enjoy!

Natural Prescription for Health: Use fresh, organic ingredients to enhance the results of your cooking effort. Add rice noodles.

Personal Thoughts/Goals:

_____

_____

_____

_____

Day 95

Proper pH

Like one who takes away a garment in cold weather, and like vinegar [acid] on soda [alkalinity]… (Proverbs 25:20).

In God's Word, mixing vinegar (which is acidic) and baking soda equals turmoil. In your body, a balanced pH is necessary to function. We evaluate all of our patients' saliva pH. Monitoring the pH level in your saliva is a noninvasive tool we use to "check the battery" and determine how the body is functioning. Fruits and vegetables shift the body toward an alkaline state. Meat, grains, and stress tilt it toward the acid side. The range for acid is from 4.5 to 7.5 for alkalinity. This corresponds with yellow to purple on nitrazine paper.

Generally I like to see the saliva pH around 6.5. There are many schools of thought on pH. Patients with a higher pH, especially females over forty, tend to have migrating pain or common shoulder bursitis pain. An alkaline, or purple color, is common in those who consume orange juice, oranges, and grapefruit (however, you should continue to eat a lemon wedge daily in water). Acid pH is found in patients who are stressed, eat meat, drink little water, and may have degenerative health problems, even cancer. The body has a natural tendency to be acid. You want to maintain a neutral value.

Natural Prescription for Health: If you have pain and drink or eat an orange or grapefruit daily, limit citrus consumption for one month.

Personal Thoughts/Goals:

_____

_____

_____

_____

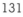

Day 96

Taste the Wonderful Stuff

Every man at the beginning sets out the good wine, and when the guests have well drunk, then the inferior. You have kept the good wine until now! (John 2:10).

Jesus saved the best for last. Everything He did was quality and with purpose. Let's turn it up a notch. The way to attract most peoples' attention is through the stomach. The "Wedding Planner" at Canaan learned a lesson—quality before quantity. In our hurry-up, fast-paced lifestyles, the art of cooking has been delegated to convenience and super-sized deli departments at grocery stores.

Let me help you a bit. Make your own food when asked to bring a dish to an event. Fresh and organic is the secret weapon. Mushrooms sliced thin hold their essence versus mushrooms from a can. Commercially preserved or packaged food is bland and limp. Pine nuts, sesame seeds, or walnuts added to a salad or vegetable enhance the protein content and taste. Celery hearts are milder than outer sticks. Lightly grate the peel of lemon for a special accent. Almond or vanilla extract blended with maple syrup over sweet potatoes and/or apples will bring people back for more. Create simple touches with meals. You will reap the benefit of knowing you shared quality food for a meal. Live it up!

Natural Prescription for Health: Add your favorite fresh herb or herbs to your salad, entrees, or side dishes instead of commercial taste enhancers.

Personal Thoughts/Goals:

_____

_____

_____

_____

Day 97

Natural Flavor Spices

Five hundred shekels of cassia [cinnamon]...*and a bin of olive oil* (Exodus 30:24).

When God created the planet He provided for us naturally all of our wants, needs, and desires. One of my favorite spices is cinnamon. The aroma of cinnamon on anything activates every smell and taste receptor in my body.

There are many ways to use organic cinnamon. Be creative. Start your day with fresh, gluten free quinoa or short grain brown rice. Add some raw almonds and a sprinkle of cinnamon. Bake some apples (leave the peel on to prevent loss of moisture and nutrients) and sprinkle some cinnamon on them when fork-tender. We make our own applesauce. It's easy. Peel, core, cut the apples into small cubes, and add a small amount of pure water to a cooking pot. Simmer on low heat until tender, smash, and cool. Sprinkle with cinnamon for flavor. Try cinnamon on brown rice or grits. For extraordinary essence, adding cinnamon to oils is a treat. Use some creative imagination.

Natural Prescription for Health: Add cinnamon to baked yams or sweet potatoes.

Personal Thoughts/Goals:

_____

_____

_____

_____

Day 98

The Best Meds

In an Italian study of 180 people with the metabolic syndrome, those who ate a healthy Mediterranean diet had less inflammation and insulin resistance.

Patients on the Mediterranean diet ate twice as much fruit, vegetables, beans, nuts, whole grains, olive oil, and Omega 3 fats (largely from fish), and half as much saturated fat as the control group. Both groups consumed roughly equal amounts of alcohol, total fat, protein, and carbohydrates.

After two years, signs of insulin resistance and inflammation (like C-reactive protein and interleukin-6) were lower, and blood vessels were more flexible in the Mediterranean dieters than in the control group.

What's more, the Mediterranean group improved more than the control group on all measures of the metabolic syndrome—large waist size, low HDL ("good") cholesterol, and higher-than-optimal blood sugar, blood pressure, and triglycerides.[17]

Natural Prescription for Health: Eat more fruits, vegetables, beans, whole grains, and seafood. Replace saturated fats from meat and dairy with unsaturated fats from oils and nuts.

> I had restricted range of motion and pain in my neck and shoulder when I first came to see Dr. DeMaria. I began consuming organic foods and reduced or eliminated dairy, hydrogenated fats, and sugar. I also implemented traction and regular spinal adjustments. Following Dr. Bob's advice and care has reduced my pain and increased my strength, energy, and range of motion. Because of the honest information available through education, the patient is inspired and encouraged to take the primary active role in his healing and health maintenance rather than being an ill, ignorant, drug-dependent lemming. —Kevin Gallagher

Personal Thoughts/Goals:

_____

_____

_____

_____

Day 99

Beet Root

I will be like the dew to Israel; he shall grow like the lily,
and lengthen his roots like Lebanon (Hosea 14:5).

L et food be your medicine, and let medicine be your food. What a profound statement.

I am constantly telling my patients the benefit of eating beets. It has been determined that even a small percentage of beet fiber in a diet with a person having high serum cholesterol can reduce it by thirty percent. Yes, you read it right, and I have the patients to prove it. The lowering of cholesterol with beet fiber is associated with the elevation of HDL cholesterol, a sign that your body is reducing inflammation.

The best way to incorporate organic beets is grated, raw on a mixed green salad. I encourage patients to eat them raw or baked. You can also cut and peel the beets to the size you would cut potatoes to be mashed. Add balsamic vinegar and a splash of coconut oil (it can handle high heat). Sprinkle with Celtic Sea Salt, cover and bake at 400 degrees for one hour. Cool; sprinkle with olive or flax oil and enjoy. Do not boil beets. Commercially canned and pickled beets are the last choice. Don't be alarmed; beets can color your stool and urine.

Natural Prescription for Health: When preparing beets, wear some type of covering on the hands to prevent staining. Latex or rubber gloves work well.

Personal Thoughts/Goals:

_____

_____

_____

_____

Day 100

Dr. Bob's Turkey Meatballs

A man's heart plans his way. But the Lord directs his steps (Proverbs 16:9).

Plan—build your life on a foundation. Convenience and simplicity are necessary commodities for busy people. Many stores today that are in touch with health conscious American appetites have selections available that are affordable and chemical free. However, I have yet to find quality turkey meatballs. The products I have found have sugar as one of the first ingredients.

I use turkey meatballs occasionally for lunch with my salad. I purchase two pounds of fresh ground turkey breast and thigh meat and mix the two blends together. Then I add a natural, organic egg, Celtic Sea Salt, bread crumbs, organic Italian herbs, freshly grated parmesan cheese, and a dash of organic catsup without sugar added. You can put any item in your recipe; flax seeds would be an interesting extra. Roll the meatballs to a medium size. You can sauté them in olive oil or bake them at 350 degrees for 40-50 minutes. Cool and freeze in a closed container. Thaw, warm, and "gobble" them up!

Natural Prescription for Health: Prepare items in advance for future meals, ground organic chicken thigh and breast can be used as a turkey substitute.

Personal Thoughts/Goals:

_____

_____

_____

_____

Day 101

Spices

If it must be so, then do this: Take…a little balm and a little honey, spices…
(Genesis 43:11).

Spices are mentioned several times throughout the Bible, starting from the beginning. Natural God-given herbs and spices add zest to food. Human-made enhancers, though, can confuse the nervous system. Monosodium glutamate (MSG) is probably the most notorious of all. If you are sensitive to MSG, common in Chinese food, it can be a sign of a vitamin B6 deficiency. Be a label reader. Texturized protein can be a stealthy, human-made taste bud supercharger. Human-made chemicals are generally toxic and interfere with natural body cycles.

Your favorite herbs and spices can be grown in your own backyard or herb box. Basil is my first choice. I use celery, dill seeds, oregano, parsley, pepper, poultry seasoning, thyme, and tumeric. I also enjoy cinnamon and ginger. My least favorites are sage and rosemary; however, you may love these flavors. Try adding herbs during the middle or at the end of cooking.

Natural Prescription for Health: Add basil and chives to your mixed green salad. Chives also taste great in egg salad sandwiches, along with safflower oil mayonnaise and Celtic Sea Salt.

Personal Thoughts/Goals:

_____

_____

_____

_____

Day 102

Dr. Bob's Cooking Secret

And make me savory food, such as I love, and bring it to me that I may eat,
that my soul may bless you before I die (Genesis 27:4).

I have a Native American friend whom I respect and from whom I have gleaned practical life applications. Jesus taught in parables and simple truths, but the educated at the time were too proud and stiff-necked to learn. They lacked love.

A secret weapon used to create a luscious meal is love. Cook with an emotional mindset of love. My friend, a certified nutritional consultant and cookbook author says, "The love permeates through the food." I enjoy making multigrain pancakes for my sons. I add little enhancers to the stack of cakes. A dash of pure vanilla stimulates taste buds along with a few drops of stevia, a natural herb sweetener. Warm organic-sourced maple syrup along with one hundred percent butter creates a lasting memory. My sons still talk about their weekend pancakes. Add love to all the meals you prepare.

Natural Prescription for Health: Organic vanilla extract can be added to any food— be creative. Plan a special meal with love.

Personal Thoughts/Goals:

_____

_____

_____

_____

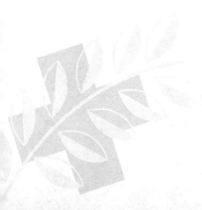

Day 103

We Use Garlic

We remember…the garlic… (Numbers 11:5).

The Israelites craved foods from Egypt—especially garlic. Garlic had medicinal properties that were not found in the "odorless" plants. It is often referred to as Chinese or even Russian penicillin.

Reality of life dictates what you are going to eat. Garlic has been found to stimulate natural protection against tumor cells. It also provides the liver with a certain amount of protection against chemicals that cause cancer. Even though garlic attacks tumor cells, it is harmless to normal, healthy body cells. Although bad breath from fresh garlic can be a little repelling, it can lower blood pressure, lower cholesterol, and cleanse the blood of impurities. Now you see why the Israelites craved garlic.

I like to roast garlic in a clay roaster. Then I squeeze the garlic flesh from the clove and spread it on bread with olive or flax oil.

Natural Prescription for Health: Roast cloves of garlic in a covered dish in one-fourth inch of water for one hour at 400 degrees. Spread on bread or add to salads and side dishes. Store in an air tight container.

Personal Thoughts/Goals:

_____

_____

_____

_____

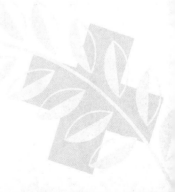

Day 104

Dr. Bob's Grill Tips

Then they shall eat the flesh on that night: roasted in fire, with unleavened bread and with bitter herbs they shall eat it (Exodus 12:8).

"*The lazy man does not roast what he took in hunting. But diligence is man's precious possession*" (Prov. 12:27). Taking the time to cook your own meals creates a level of personal satisfaction and accomplishment. My mouth waters when I drive along during spring and summer taking in the sizzling aroma of roasted barbecue. I enjoy grilling. I normally grill chicken at a medium setting using a gas grill and add poultry seasoning along with Celtic Sea Salt. Sometimes I prebake chicken with onion and celery, usually one-half hour at 350 degrees, covered.

You can make your own barbecue sauce with sugar-free catsup, chili sauce, and maple syrup or honey. Brush it on with a paint brush while cooking over low heat. Tenderloin meats (beef, lamb, or turkey) are juicy when first grilled at an extremely high temperature to create an outer crust, keeping the juice inside, then lowering the heat to cook thoroughly. I also grill vegetables; brushing on olive oil after they have warmed 10 or 15 minutes. Grilled onions with olive oil are a nice extra side dish.

Natural Prescription for Health: Season fresh meat with Celtic Sea Salt, poultry seasoning, or Italian dressing. The cooked items will keep for a few days, stored in air tight containers.

Personal Thoughts/Goals:

_____

_____

_____

_____

Day 105

See More, Eat More

The larger the serving size, the more you're likely to eat, says a study from Pennsylvania State University. Researchers told fifty-one men and women in their twenties to eat as much macaroni and cheese as they wanted at a no-cost lunch. It didn't matter if they were male or female, overweight or trim. When the portions (either on their plates or on a serving dish) were large (thirty-five ounces), on average they ate about thirty percent more calories than when the portions were smaller (eighteen ounces). What's more, the people reported feeling no fuller after eating the big portions than the smaller ones.[18]

Natural Prescription for Health: If you're trying to cut calories, shrink your servings. Some suggestions: Order a small portion, split a dish with someone, or stash half of what you're served in a doggie bag before you start eating.

> When I first came to see Dr. DeMaria, I had been dealing with upper and lower back pain. After following Dr. Bob's advice, I cut back on sweets and fried foods, and I am trying to cut back on dairy. It has been difficult not giving in to cravings for sugar and dairy, but I now know how the food I eat affects my body. I have also begun taking supplements, and I exercise more often. I really enjoy how the Word of God is discussed so openly in the office, and I feel that Dr. and Mrs. DeMaria are really in this business because they truly care and want to help people. —Jane Zilka

Personal Thoughts/Goals:

_____

_____

_____

_____

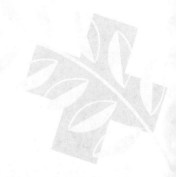

Meal Debriefing

The Meal Assessment Guide is a template of eating patterns that I use when consulting with my patients. The purpose of the questions is to create a mindset of foods that may create digestive distress and/or pain. Certain foods, regardless of media hype or conventional thinking established by food manufacturers, may initiate your downward health condition.

The information I have presented is based on real clinical experience with positive results. Many meal suggestions that you read in magazines, newspapers, or on the Internet are placed there by the industry that has the most to win financially. I can guarantee you this—breakfasts consisting of yogurt, bananas, and cereal; lunches consisting of burgers and fries; and dinners that include pasta, cream sauces, and dessert will precipitate pain.

See the Transition Chart for a simple progression to a diet that promotes pain-free tissues and joints.

Transition Chart

The following is an excellent transition chart to help you make a smooth transition to eating healthier foods. This information was taken in part from, *Junk Food to Real Food, A Blueprint for Healthier Eating*, by Carol A. Nostrand.[19]

Foods to Avoid Proteins	Foods to Enjoy Proteins	
Eliminate Immediately	*Acceptable Foods Experiment with these:*	*Vital Foods Primarily use these:*
Meats with additives, such as luncheon meat packed with nitrites (bologna, salami, etc.)	Meat without additives, hormones, antibiotics, etc., raised free-range on organic feed	Sprouts
		Fresh, raw nuts and seeds: flax, chia, pumpkin, sunflower, sesame, almond, pecan, brazil, walnut, filbert, etc.
Meat with hormones, etc.	Deep ocean or pure-lake fish	
Processed cheese		Nut butters
Processed eggs	Nuts and grains as the source to make rice, almond milk, cheese, and yogurt	Nut milks
Processed chicken (raised in small coops, injected with antibiotics, etc.)		Organic eggs
Pork	Goat's milk, chevre, feta cheese (goat's milk is very close to human milk constituents) is acceptable, but not daily	Beans: lentils, split peas, black beans, etc.
Pasteurized, homogenized cow's milk		Tofu, tempeh (No Genetic Modified, focus on organic sourced soy)
Yogurt with sugar, and toxic additives		

Foods to Avoid **Carbohydrates**	**Foods to Enjoy** **Carbohydrates**	
Eliminate *Immediately*	*Acceptable Foods* *Experiment with these:*	*Vital Foods* *Primarily use these:*
Sugar: white, brown, turbinado, sucrose, glucose, corn syrup, fructose, etc.	Raw honey, blackstrap molasses, barley malt, pure maple syrup	Vegetables: squash, carrots, celery, tomatoes, beets, cabbage, broccoli, cauliflower, leeks, turnips, radish, lettuce, etc.
Chocolate	Carob	
Processed carbohydrates such as white flour and white flour products	Whole-grain bread Whole-grain pasta	Fruit: apples, pears, plums, etc.
White rice	Grain/nut ice cream made without toxic additives or sugar	Sea vegetables
Anything packaged or canned with sugar, salt or toxic additives		Whole grains: brown rice, millet, rye, barley, etc.
Processed pasta		
Ice cream with sugar and toxic additives		
Foods to Avoid **Lipids**	**Foods to Enjoy** **Lipids**	
Eliminate *Immediately*	*Acceptable Foods* *Experiment with these:*	*Vital Foods* *Primarily use these:*
Oils that are rancid or overheated	High oleic safflower, sunflower, olive oil	Raw, cold-processed oils: olive, sunflower, sesame, flax, almond, walnut, avocado
Rancid animal fats, such as lard, bacon drippings, etc.	Butter	Raw, unsalted butter
Anything deep-fat fried		Avocado
Artificially hardened fats, such as margarine and shortenings		Fresh, raw nuts and seeds

Foods to Avoid Other	Foods to Enjoy Other	
Eliminate Immediately	*Acceptable Foods Experiment with these:*	*Vital Foods Primarily use these:*
Coffee, tannic-acid teas, excess alcohol	Pure grain coffee substitutes	Herb teas and seasonings
Common table salt (sodium chloride)	Not more than one glass a day of non-chemicalized wine or beer	Organic apple cider vinegar
Any commercial condiments with sugar, salt or toxic additives	Aluminum-free baking powder	Homemade condiments without salt or sugar
Commercial soft drinks made with toxic additives and sugar	Soft drinks made without chemicals, sugar or toxic additives	Freshly juiced vegetables and fruits
	Potassium-balanced salt, Celtic Sea Salt	Fresh fruit ice cream
	Vegetable salt and kelp	Reverse osmosis purified water

A Comment About Soy

The more I read, study, and observe my patients, especially females, I notice decreased breast tenderness and decreased heavy menstrual flow with a reduction in soy products. If you have a question about soy in your diet, you may want to minimize it for three months and monitor your own body function. Soy products from my experience may interfere with normal thyroid function. Always discuss your health conditions with your healthcare provider.

Designing Dinner

Keep food consumption light in the evening. Focus on veggies and light protein. Eating carbohydrates, including pasta, grains, and rice, may stimulate evening cravings. You can use turkey and chicken as an animal protein base. Meatballs, meatloaf, and stir-fry are easy. Plant proteins including beans and legumes mix better with starches. Squash, such as butternut or acorn, are complex carbohydrates that affect blood sugar slowly and are best if eaten alone.

As a part of the last week of this pattern, you will have the opportunity to record and assess your dinner habits.

New research and technology may alter your strategy for eating. I would suggest you journal what you eat for at least one month if you contend with sinus issues, skin challenges, pain syndromes, and bowel dysfunction; these systems are impacted by food and the environment. The saying "one man's passion is another man's poison" has to do with what you are putting in and on your body. In the ever-changing world of toxic chemicals used as herbicides and pesticides compounded with the unwise acceptance of genetically-engineered or modified food, you would do your best to keep up with the latest research from independent sources (that is, information not presented by the food manufactures). I continually learn new physiology that helps me treat chronic health challenges in my patients without drugs or medications, whether prescription or over-the-counter. Common foods of days gone by have been altered or tampered with and actually may be a part of your health puzzle; you may want to assess your intake of gluten foods—barley, wheat, rye, and oats. Also be aware that nightshades can create your distress—tomatoes, white potatoes, eggplant, green peppers, paprika, peanuts, ashwaganda, and hot peppers. Vegans and vegetarians may have questions about meat products; be aware of your sources and quality of protein; organic everything is critically important.

Resist dessert.

Day 106

"What Can I Eat?"

*And out of the ground the Lord God made every tree grow that
is pleasant to the sight and good for food* (Genesis 2:9).

You can eat anything you want—as long as it rots. We live in a toxic environment. People, in their ignorance, have created food items that have a long shelf life, increasing profits but decreasing healthiness.

Use God's wisdom when choosing food to eat. The recommendations found in Leviticus 11 and 12 promote life. They are not there to punish you but to save you from having "body breakdown." Paul shared a profound statement in First Corinthians 6:12, *"All things are lawful for me, but all things are not helpful."* Please meditate on that statement prior to going grocery shopping or eating out.

Eat food that you prepare from living, whole food ingredients, preferably organic. Cravings for sugar will diminish over time when you fill your system with quality complex carbohydrates followed by plant-based proteins like almonds, walnuts, and other nuts.

Natural Prescription for Health: God made food without chemicals to fuel the system. Human-made food causes the machine (you) to misfire and get sick!

Personal Thoughts/Goals:

_____

_____

_____

_____

Day 107

The Oldest Grain

If a man dedicates to the Lord part of a field of his possession,
then your valuation shall be according to the seed for it. A homer of barley
seed shall be valued at fifty shekels of silver (Leviticus 27:16).

Barley was very important in days gone by, if you suspect a gluten sensitivity you may want to avoid barley; caramel coloring common in soda and "brown" bread may be sourced from barley. You do not hear too much about barley in America these days. Wheat appears to have taken over as the primary grain. During the plagues in Egypt, barley was destroyed by a hailstorm. Jesus fed the multitude with a start of five barley loaves and two fishes. Barley is one of those foods, like squash, that is easy to grow, but it is not a part of our culture. It is a heavy starch best eaten alone or with vegetables. Buy a bag and read the cooking directions. Sprinkle with your favorite herb and eat it as a main dish. Barley is very filling. You can even add some almonds for protein. It's also great in vegetable soups.

By the way, butternut squash is one of the easiest and tastiest dishes to make. Set your oven at 350 degrees. Spray olive oil on the bottom of a glass baking dish. Cut the butternut squash in half. Add a touch of water and cover. Bake 45 minutes or until tender. Serve hot with olive oil. Very good!

Natural Prescription for Health: Use barley instead of rice or potatoes.

Personal Thoughts/Goals:

_____

_____

_____

_____

Day 108

"Where's the Beef?"

*And you shall do to Ai and its king as you did to Jericho and its king. Only its spoil and its **cattle** you shall take as booty for yourselves…* (Joshua 8:2, emphasis added).

Beef is healthy, especially if you focus on the flesh and not the cover fat. Overfeeding and overmedicating commercial animal tissue with hormones and antibiotics have altered what God made for good. Beef was *not* one of the forbidden foods in the Bible.

Beef has a variety of fats, not just saturated fats, which have been associated with stiff, hard blood vessels. I do not eat beef every day. Attempt to obtain beef from a natural, organic source. Chemical-free, grass-fed beef is a good source of Omega 3 fats. Pork is not to be classified with beef.

I generally avoid eating beef when I am out for dinner. You need to be aware of the tenderizers and sources of flavor additives used to flavor your favorite dishes. I have found by trial and error that when I have eaten beef at a restaurant and wake up hot, sweaty, or thirsty, I know my body is working overtime to process the chemical tenderizer assault. We use a pressure cooker to make several of our beef dishes. You do not lose nutrients in pressure cooking like you do with other methods.

Natural Prescription for Health: Pressure-cook lean, organic beef; it's great added to stir-fried vegetables.

Personal Thoughts/Goals:

_____

_____

_____

_____

Day 109

Aspirin Death Sentence

Then Joshua called for them, and he spoke to them, saying, "Why have you deceived us…"
(Joshua 9:22).

This may be a huge shock to some of you, but taking an aspirin every day is not normal or natural. You are putting a chemical in your body that is altering or changing how your cells were designed to work. These are the questions: Why does your body need it? What is wrong? The theory is that if your blood is thin you are more likely to survive a heart attack. But why? What caused your blood to get thick like sludge with red blood cells sticking together? If you could prevent thick blood, would you need the aspirin? What happened?

Do you know you can die from taking aspirin? Aspirin can thin your blood too much. You can get ulcers or have a stroke, and even fractures heal more slowly with aspirin use. The aspirin makers lead people to believe that it is a vitamin, but aspirin can actually cause liver and kidney disease. The American public has been deceived. What you eat, drink, and smoke causes inflammation. Sugar, dairy, too much red meat, trans fat, and soda create an inflammatory state in your blood vessels. Focus on flax oil and olive oil, brown rice syrup in baked goods, almond, rice or coconut milk, chicken, turkey, fish, and herbal tea or water. Eat fresh vegetables daily.

Natural Prescription for Health: Avoid overeating inflammation-producing sugar and dairy products.

Personal Thoughts/Goals:

_____

_____

_____

_____

Day 110

All Natural

How the animals groan! The herds of cattle are restless, because they have no pasture...
(Joel 1:18).

God created people to have dominion over the fish in the sea, birds in the air, and animals in the pasture. I encourage consumption of meat products from a natural, pure source. How an animal is handled affects the taste. You want the animal raised so its natural immunity is enhanced. Calves should spend their first eight to ten months with their mother. The mother's milk has natural antibodies ensuring wellness without antibiotics. Look for sources of beef that are not fed other animal by-products. By feeding animals a well-balanced, nutritional diet with grass, the producers are able to avoid the use of unnatural digestive aids commonly used in conventional cattle production. Range-fed beef with extra room to grow affects the texture and quality. I can taste the difference in various meat sources.

Does the beef, chicken, turkey, or lamb you eat cause digestive distress? It may be the chemicals given to the animals. Do some research; there are excellent sources of safe animal tissue.

Natural Prescription for Health: Evaluate your digestive response to any animal tissue you consume. Vary sources if you experience distress. Be mindful of marinated products.

Personal Thoughts/Goals:

_____

_____

_____

_____

Day 111

Safe Fish?

Everything in the waters that has not fins or scales shall be abhorrent and detestable to you (Leviticus 11:12 AMP).

Fish is an excellent source of protein and fat essential for optimum brain function. Old Testament dietary instructions are as significant today as in the time of Moses. "…You may eat any fish that have fins and scales…You are to detest all others" (see Lev. 11:9-10). Scales can be removed without tearing the fish skin. Fish that are considered unclean are swordfish, shark, lumpfish, and European flatfish. These also have the highest levels of mercury and pesticides.

Another group of scaleless fish include crustacean and mollusk shellfish. This includes clams, mussels, oysters, scallops, shrimp, and lobster. These are considered "scavenger feeders" that clean their environment. The poisons from this process stay in the flesh of the shellfish and are a major source of poison to humans.

Natural Prescription for Health: Deep water ocean fish are excellent sources of Omega 3 fat. Avoid farm-raised fish.

Personal Thoughts/Goals:

_____

_____

_____

_____

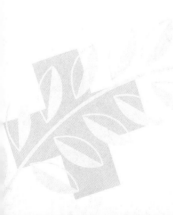

Day 112

Seafood & Stroke

Men who ate seafood at least once a month were roughly forty percent less likely to have an ischemic stroke than men who ate seafood less often in a study of more than forty-three thousand health professionals. Ischemic strokes are caused by clogged arteries. Fish-eaters had no lower risk of strokes caused by hemorrhage (which occurred about a quarter as often). Eating seafood more than once a month didn't lower the risk further.[20]

Natural Prescription for Health: Eat seafood at least once or twice a week if possible. (You may only need one serving a month to reduce your risk of stroke, but earlier studies suggested that eating one or two servings a week can reduce your risk of heart disease.) If you don't eat fish, try to add flax oil to boost your intake of alpha-linolenic acid, which your body may convert to the Omega 3 fats that are in fish oil. While this study offered a hint that alpha-linolenic acid may protect against strokes, it's too early to say for sure.

> I had eczema on my hands and feet along with very sore, achy joints. I also had almost constant headaches. I took Tylenol (or other NSAIDS) almost daily, sometimes two or three times a day. The information and care provided by Dr. DeMaria has improved my life. My hands and feet are almost completely cleared up. I have stopped eating red meat, white potatoes, caffeine, chocolate, sugar, wheat, and tomatoes, and I have started eating more fresh veggies, fresh fruit, and fish. Remembering to drink my water on busy days has been the most difficult for me. —Ginny Evans

Personal Thoughts/Goals:

_____

_____

_____

_____

Day 113

Who Is Guiding Your Ship?

*…No longer be children tossed to and fro and carried about with
every wind of doctrine, by the **trickery** of men…*
(Ephesians 4:14, emphasis added).

God wants us to present our bodies a living sacrifice, holy, acceptable to God *"which is your reasonable service. And do not be conformed to this world, but be transformed by the renewing of your mind…"* (Rom. 12:1-2). This is a mandate to keep your body in good, working order. Allow God to be the guide of your ship. Look to His Word for direction.

In the beginning of God's Word, we are advised to eat living food with seed. My advice to you is to eat whole food such as broccoli, cabbage, green and yellow beans, squash, celery—real food. Jesus also ate lamb, figs, fish, and bread. I suggest that, even in your hectic life, you plan your meals ahead of time, focusing on the use of organic items. No plan is a plan to fail.

Don't be tricked into believing that processed food is wholesome. Try something new, for example: ground turkey thigh and breast mixed with an organic egg, sugar-free catsup, bread crumbs, and Italian herbs. Press into a baking dish and cover. Bake at 350 degrees for one hour or until tender and brown. Slice and freeze. Take slices out on days when you are pressed for time. This is a delicious fast-food substitute when combined with your favorite sauce, in salads, or eaten alone.

Natural Prescription for Health: Plan and purchase products to create one week of meals.

Personal Thoughts/Goals:

_____

_____

_____

_____

Day 114

What Came With Dinner?

Then immediately an angel of the Lord struck him, because he did not give glory to God. And he was eaten by **worms** *and died* (Acts 12:23, emphasis added).

This may be news to some of you—parasites are a common cause of many health conditions. Americans do not like to accept the fact that we have parasites living inside our bodies. But it has been estimated that there are more parasitic infections acquired in this country (the United States) than in Africa. According to a study reported in *Health Quarters Monthly* (Vol. 77, March 2005), approximately seventy-nine million Americans have parasite infestation.

Sushi, which is found in many grocery stores and restaurants, can be the source of parasites or worms—some growing up to forty feet long. A diet high in refined carbohydrates, or sugar, supplying few nutrients, increases a person's susceptibility to infestation. When a person is afflicted with parasites, the body's supply of nutrients is depleted to the point that supplementation of all nutrients is necessary to restore normal health. We use a natural enzyme and sulfur product to control parasite growth. Parasites do not like sulfur sourced naturally from eggs, onion, garlic and cruciferous veggies.

Natural Prescription for Health: Completely cook all food. Do not eat raw meat or fish.

Personal Thoughts/Goals:

_____

_____

_____

_____

Day 115

One Food at a Time

While dining with a ruler [someone significant in your life], *pay attention to what is put before you* (Proverbs 23:2 NLT).

Do you suffer with digestive distress? Do you have a relentless, gnawing pain in the pit of your stomach that creates fear and anxiety and interferes with life? Timothy suffered with digestive distress. A leading, missed cause of digestive pain is eating different food in layers that the body is not capable of processing. One such example is starch. Starchy veggies and grains are best eaten alone, *not* with animal protein. Protein needs an acid environment; potatoes are best digested with alkaline. Putting the two together stops or slows digestion. When digestion stops, putrefaction starts, extra inorganic acid is made, and you have pain.

My recommendation is to try eating starches alone or with greens and veggies (see Food Combination charts, pages 119–120). It is best to eat meat alone, not with starch or with veggies. The all-American fast food staple, burger-bread-and-fries, inevitably will lead to digestive pain.

If you are a big eater, try a little self-control and skip all the delicacies after your meal. Deception may be involved. Steven Covey says, "If you cannot control your appetite, can you control other emotions?"

Natural Prescription for Health: Eat starches and greens alone, not in combination with other foods.

Personal Thoughts/Goals:

_____

_____

_____

_____

Day 116

Eat in Peace

Better is a dinner of herbs where love is, than a fatted calf with hatred
(Proverbs 15:17).

God's Word encourages you to eat your morsels of food in peace without distress. Chew your food long and slowly. This will reduce the amount of work your stomach and pancreas need to do. Eating food fast and furiously will create digestive distress and inhibit liver function. The liver and pancreas contribute bile and enzymes to the food bolus. Emotional distress can impair the release of these natural digestive aides resulting in malabsorption.

As mentioned previously, you are what you eat and absorb. People in duress appear to look and feel unhealthy. They may even lose weight during times of trial and tribulation. You may be eating and not utilizing. Do you have family and personal issues to be rectified? Slowly, diplomatically create an environment around the dinner table that encourages quiet, logical, and loving conversation. In our home, we make dinnertime a healthy priority. Take a step toward establishing family dinnertime.

Natural Prescription for Health: Do not eat while you are on the run in your car. Always take time to break bread around the table—even if it is only one healthy, fast food meal a day.

Personal Thoughts/Goals:

_____

_____

_____

_____

Day 117

Stir-Fry

So Gideon went in and prepared a young goat, and unleavened bread from an ephah of flour. The meat he put in a basket, and he put the broth in a pot... (Judges 6:19).

Stir-fry meals are simple, easy, and healthy, depending on what you choose to prepare. Purchase a wok that is electric or one that can be warmed on top of the stove. Plan ahead when you shop. Purchase one- or two-pound packages of organic chicken, turkey, fish, squid, or beef pieces. You can sift wheat, rice, oat, or barley flour on the meat and brown it with olive oil. Add bean sprouts, snow peas, onion, celery, eggplant pieces, water chestnuts, cabbage, cashews, small corn cobs, broccoli, and any vegetable you like.

Purchase organic vegetable broth as a base. We use the product Shari Ann's, which can be purchased at most health food stores. There is a wheat free soy sauce called Organic Tamari made by San-J. I also add sesame seeds, Celtic Sea Salt, and fresh herbs such as basil, chives, and parsley. Simmer over medium heat, cooking until tender. Simultaneously prepare flat rice noodles.

Natural Prescription for Health: Plan a stir fry meal—a handy way to clean out your refrigerator. This is a healthy alternative to any fast food. Consider avoiding nightshade veggies and gluten-based flours in all meal planning, including stir-frying, if you continue to chronically experience pain, skin problems, headache, fatigue, fibromyalgia, or digestive symptoms.

Personal Thoughts/Goals:

_____

_____

_____

_____

Day 118

Body Fertilizer

*A certain man had a fig tree planted in his vineyard, and he came seeking
fruit on it and found none. ... "Sir, let it alone this year also, until
I dig around it and fertilize it"* (Luke 13:6,8).

Creation requires nutrients to thrive. Trees, plants, herbs, flowers, grasses and any type of living, growing seed or fruit-producing vegetation requires food and water. We need to "fertilize" our physical bodies in these stressful, time-pressed days. Poor quality and overworked soil produces inferior vegetation and low-quality edible by-products. I encourage patients to avoid conventionally-grown fruits and vegetables. You can taste the difference.

Recently, while I was teaching a group of doctors, "seminar food" was served. The salad was tasteless, and the fish, chicken, and veggies did not have the zest found in organic food. The experience was such that my bowels were affected. I know now why our society is plagued with health issues.

Quality food is your fertilizer. Don't cook food to death. Avoid synthetic vitamins. Focus on quality ingredients in your food. I use whole food and cold-processed supplements that I recommend to patients only after I survey their body signals and evaluate their food journal.

Natural Prescription for Health: Not feeling at peak performance? Journal food patterns for one week. Wheat, corn, dairy, sugar, nightshades, alcohol, and citrus are common energy zappers. Look at the labels of all fruits and vegetables. A PLU number on the label starting with 9 indicates organic, and an 8 indicates genetically-engineered. All other numbers are considered conventional, which means they have herbicides and pesticides.

Personal Thoughts/Goals:

_____

_____

_____

_____

Day 119

Mediterranean Mix

In a study of more than twenty-two thousand adults in Greece, those who ate a more traditional Mediterranean diet had a lower death rate (largely due to fewer deaths from heart disease and cancer) than others. Participants received points for eating foods like vegetables, fruits, beans, fish, and olive oil more often and for eating foods like meat and dairy products (which are rarely low-fat in Greece) less often. They also received points for consuming moderate amounts of alcohol. A lower death rate wasn't linked to any single food group.[21]

Natural Prescription for Health: It's possible that something else about the people who chose to eat a Mediterranean diet kept them alive longer. But there's plenty of evidence from other studies to recommend less fatty meat and dairy and more vegetables, fruits, beans, fish, and unsaturated oils like olive and canola.

> I had aches in my back and legs along with stomach discomfort when I first came to see Dr. DeMaria. The adjustments have improved my posture and the massage therapy has improved my gait. The recommended diet modifications have been the most difficult. I love sweet things. I eventually hope to get off Lipitor and Celebrex completely. My wife finds me easier to get along with since beginning my visits here. —Ted Lang

Personal Thoughts/Goals:

_____

_____

_____

_____

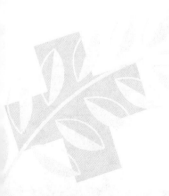

Day 120

Drugless Care

...The head—Christ—from whom the whole body, joined and knit together by what every joint supplies, according to the effective working by which every part does its share, causes growth of the body for the edifying of itself in love (Ephesians 4:15-16).

How would you like to get healthy and stay healthy without medication? Sound farfetched? It's not. An ounce of prevention is worth a pound of cure. Common conditions requiring medical assistance including antibiotics or pain relievers can be traced to what is being eaten and, over time, toxic accumulation. Choose items with complex-based sweeteners like brown rice syrup or the herb stevia. Drink water. Recently, a patient told me how significant changing from processed food with herbicides and pesticides to fresh, organic meals totally changed her health. She assumed not feeling one hundred percent was normal—until she changed what she ate.

Nervous system misfires are a stealth factor in even the most chronic conditions. Communication from the brain cells to tissue cells is a part of the 24/7 monitoring system that works automatically unless it is altered due to compressed nerve tissue by vertebral misplacement. Regular spinal assessment is a logical adjunct to optimal health.

Natural Prescription for Health: Consume less conventional, processed food and focus on organic food.

Personal Thoughts/Goals:

_____

_____

_____

Dinner Journal:

_____

_____

_____

Day 121

Beans

[They] *brought beds and basins, earthen vessels and wheat, barley and flour, parched grain and beans…* (2 Samuel 17:28).

We have been blessed with a wide variety of foods. Diversification is a wise approach. Avoid eating the same choices all the time.

I normally do not eat lentils, but they can easily be incorporated as a side or main dish. I normally eat string green or yellow beans. They are a source of vitamins, minerals, iron, Omega 3 fat, and protein. I like to clean the ends of beans and blanch them in boiling water for a minute or two, cool them, and add to a mixed green salad. They will also stay crisp in an airtight container. Another suggestion is to steam beans until crisp tender (3 to 4 minutes), add sesame seeds, olive oil, Celtic Sea Salt, and chopped roasted red peppers to make a great side dish.

Organic black beans in a can are a great source of fiber and vegetable protein, which can easily be added to a mixed green salad. Lima beans mixed with yellow corn and onions along with a dash of Paul Newman's Oil and Vinegar dressing creates a colorful side dish. Create a new mindset of options.

Natural Prescription for Health: Add some beans to your salad or as a side dish!

Personal Thoughts/Goals:

_____

_____

_____

_____

Dinner Journal:

_____

_____

_____

_____

Day 122

Dr. Bob's Fatted Fowl Turkey Recipe

Now Solomon's provision for one day was…oxen…sheep…deer, gazelles, roebucks, and fatted fowl (1 Kings 4:22-23).

The first Thanksgiving apparently had roots from God's Word. I happen to be the official turkey chef in our home, and I would like to pass on a few tips. We purchase fresh, organic twelve- to twenty-pound birds, and I clean the inside of the bird thoroughly. We purchase a wheat-based, organic stuffing, and I never stuff the cavity the night before. The first thing in the morning, I boil the heart, neck, and gizzard in pure water. Then I add the flavored broth to the herbed bread stuffing; the celery and onions that have been sautéed in olive oil and one-half stick of butter; and large organic egg. Most stuffing mixes suggest adding water only. The flavored broth, egg, onion, and celery, especially moistened to wet and soft, create a flavor that will be absorbed by the turkey breast. I fill the neck and abdominal cavities with dressing and cover the openings with bread crust. I secure it with bamboo skewers and cook in an oven bag with a thermometer. An electric knife is the easiest way for me to carve the turkey when it's done.

Natural Prescription for Health: Baking a netted, boned, turkey roast is an easy-to-prepare weekend meal. Insert pieces of celery and onion into the roast for added flavor.

Personal Thoughts/Goals:

_____

_____

_____

_____

Dinner Journal:

_____

_____

_____

_____

Day 123

How God Heals

And they did not repent of their murders or their sorceries... (Revelation 9:21).

Sorceries: Generally described as the use of medicine or drugs[22]

God designed our bodies to eat and eliminate. When you make a decision to eat a food item that does not promote optimal health, do not fret too much. It will be eliminated. Matthew 15:17 says, *"Do you not yet understand that whatever enters the mouth goes into the stomach and is eliminated?"* However, continued consumption of toxic food substances eventually will lead to a state of poor health. The body will absorb nutrients from whatever you consume. Do not be fooled. Continued inappropriate choices will result in auto-intoxification, which actually means you've put yourself in a state of toxicity. Some common body signals include sinusitis, ear wax, diarrhea, colitis, skin rashes, acne, arthritis, asthma, psoriasis, pain, kidney failure, liver disease, and eye disease.

Do you get the point? Many, if not most, modern health conditions are a result of toxicity. Here is the million-dollar question: Do you take an antihistamine or pain pill to mask the symptoms of poor choices, or do you make life-enhancing decisions? Pharmaceuticals do not cure. They modify symptoms. What a smoke screen!

Natural Prescription for Health: Avoid toxic, processed food.

Personal Thoughts/Goals:

_____

_____

_____

Dinner Journal:

_____

_____

_____

Day 124

Don't Be Foolish!

But the natural man does not receive the things of the Spirit of God, for they are foolishness to him; nor can he know them, because they are spiritually discerned (1 Corinthians 2:14).

Was Christopher Columbus foolish? Certainly not! Einstein created a mathematical reasoning tool. Edison had thousands of inventions. Foolish?

Today we have advanced technology that creates a fake sense of security that can be "foolish"—causing us to believe that a pill will relieve all of the abuse caused by our lifestyle choices. Sometimes it is easy to be confused. Margarine is not a food, and aspirin is not a vitamin. Soda is loaded with chemicals, especially phosphoric acid, that can lead to osteoporosis and cavities. God created eggs as an excellent source of protein. Artificial "heart-healthy Egg Beaters" confuse the system. Processed cheese does not mold in the sun. White enriched bread will never be as good as whole wheat. Cow's milk is for cows; human milk is for humans.

Do not eat food that does not rot. Read Leviticus chapter 11. Old Covenant truths are applicable today—God-given principles never change.

Natural Prescription for Health: Say "no thank you" to social event invitations where there will be alcohol and processed foods served. Do not say, "I don't eat that."

Personal Thoughts/Goals:

_____

_____

_____

Dinner Journal:

_____

_____

_____

Day 125

Dr. Bob's Supper

*There they made Him a supper; and Martha served, but Lazarus was
one of those who sat at the table with Him* (John 12:2).

WWDBE…What Would Dr. Bob Eat? I am asked all the time, what do you eat? Well, I do eat some of what Jesus ate, such as lamb and fish. However, I don't eat figs, fruit of the vine, and I limit my bread consumption. I never eat processed food or pork. Jesus walked a lot. I run daily.

Planning is the key component for eating at home. Generally, I focus on vegetables and protein. I grill on a gas burner or a George Foreman Grill. I brush chicken, turkey, or duck with Paul Newman's Oil and Vinegar Dressing and wrap with large lettuce leaves. I place the wrap on the grill—the leaves keep the food moist. Asparagus is awesome on the grill, brushed with olive oil. We also cut up and cook onions with olive oil on the grill.

I eat steamed broccoli, carrots, and cauliflower sprinkled with sesame seeds and olive oil. You can use a bamboo or stainless steel steamer. Green beans with almonds are delicious. It is best to avoid potatoes and pasta—I do eat them but not often. Eating starch, grains, and pastas is like setting paper on fire. You always need to add fuel. Consistent carbs that are not burned create a fat reserve. Bake a rolled and boned turkey roast, but avoid deep frying.

Natural Prescription for Health: Protein is similar to adding a log to the fire. Stoke your fire with nuts and lean meat/fish.

Personal Thoughts/Goals:

_____

_____

Dinner Journal:

_____

_____

Day 126

The Dairy Diet Myth

"Drink milk...Lose weight" say the ads. The dairy industry has created an entire "Healthy Weight with Milk" campaign to boost sales. What's the evidence? Most of it came from a researcher who has a patent on the claim that dairy foods aid weight loss.

In a study—the largest so far—a high-dairy diet did not help people lose weight. Twenty-three obese patients on 1,500-calorie diets who were randomly assigned to consume four servings of dairy a day lost no more weight or body fat after six months than twenty-two others who consumed one serving a day.[23]

Natural Prescription for Health: Low-fat (or nonfat) milk, yogurt, and cheese can help lower blood pressure and boost calcium intake. But don't expect them to keep you slim.

> When I first came to see Dr. DeMaria, I was unable to lose weight. Following
> Dr. Bob's recommendations, I have eliminated soda, and I no longer add
> sugar to my coffee. I now read labels to avoid foods with hydrogenated oil,
> and I have added beets to my diet. Since making my lifestyle modifications,
> I am now able to sleep better; I have lost some weight, and I have a stronger
> back and better posture. —Julie Mead

Personal Thoughts/Goals:

_____

_____

_____

_____

Dinner Journal:

_____

_____

_____

_____

Self-Assessment
Dinner Debriefing

Using the information you wrote in your Dinner Journals, answer the following questions and mark your score as directed. Your goal is a score of five.

_____ Did you have light, late afternoon/evening dinners? Add one.

_____ Did you focus on fish, animal, or plant protein? Add one.

_____ Did you concentrate on pastas, white rice, or wheat-based items? Subtract one.

_____ Did you eat steamed, raw, or lightly sautéed vegetables? Add one.

_____ What beverage did you drink? If water, water with lemon, herbal tea (four ounces total), no change. If you drank more than four ounces of any beverage with the meal, subtract one.

_____ Did you eat at home with friends or family? Add one.

_____ Did you eat in your vehicle? Subtract one.

_____ Did you use flax or olive oil? Add one.

_____ Did you use partially hydrogenated or trans fat? Subtract one.

_____ Did you end the meal with fruit or dessert? Subtract one.

_____ Did you blend animal protein with a grain or starch? Subtract one.

_____ Did you use a sugar substitute? Subtract one.

_____ Did you eat a pork product or fish without scales, i.e., shrimp, lobster? Subtract one.

_____ Did you use condiments, relishes, or sauces with sugar or chemical enhancers? Subtract one.

_____ Total score

Dr. Bob's dinner comment: Your goal is to eat a light, late afternoon or evening meal focusing on the mid-level glycemic range (see Glycemic Foods chart, pages 171–174). Combine foods accurately. Overloading the digestive system can create liver, gallbladder, and stomach distress (see Food Combination charts, pages 119–120).

I have successfully helped patients with chronic conditions by suggesting they have a food sensitivity or IGg4 blood spot test. We look at about thirty foods when evaluating the "blood spot" specimen. You can complete requirements for this test with a simple kit, which is sent to a lab. I have discovered most patients and worldwide clients literally have digestive distress in their intestines permitting undigested food particles to be transported in the blood and lymph systems. The protein particles from the undigested foods create an alarm, and the patient suffers with histamine reactions including stuffy runny noses, headache, lung congestion, loose stools, and pain syndromes, even memory issues and fatigue. You are what you eat and digest.

Sweets and Desserts

There are times when you will crave or want something sweet. Chromium supplementation reduces the sugar desire. Protein helps keep blood sugar levels steady without fluctuations. Organic raisins are an alternative to candy.

Avoid a consistent diet of sweet fruit and snacks. They can cause pain by stressing the organ that makes natural cortisone, the adrenal gland.

Fats and Sweeteners

Fat: Gives taste to food. Every cell membrane is made of fat. Fat is necessary for brain function, heart health, and pain relief.

Saturated Fat: Found primarily in red meat. Also in coconut and palm oil. Plant oils do not have cholesterol. Saturated animal fat hardens. There are no double bonds in the chemical structure.

Monounsaturated Fat: Liquid at room temperature. Will harden when cool. There is a double bond. Excellent cooking oil with moderate temperatures. Olive oil is my favorite and most cost effective.

Polyunsaturated Oil: Liquid at all times. Can be used to heat at higher temperatures. Safflower and sunflower oils are the best choices. I normally do not eat fried foods.

Essential Fats: There are two—Omega 3 and Omega 6—and they are both necessary for optimal health life. The Omega 3 fat is commonly deficient in the standard American diet. I encourage consuming flax oil, greens, and walnuts as a source of Omega 3 fat. Do not heat flax oil. The Omega 6 oil is found in most snack foods—look for ingredients including safflower and sunflower oil. Salmon oil is a direct source of Omega 3 fats. I do not recommend long-term use unless there is monitoring of your blood coagulation (hardening time), or PT time. Omega 3 fat can improve brain function and reduce pain.

Trans Fat: Polyunsaturated fat, heated with hydrogen added. It disrupts cell membrane activity. Trans fat causes pain and raises cholesterol. Also known as partially-hydrogenated. Avoid at all times.

Glycemic Foods

(Figure 4)

It is best to choose food with glycemic indices of fifty to eighty. Foods in this range give the best chance to minimize exaggerated insulin responses.

FOOD	GLYCEMIC INDEX
Breads	
Rye (crisp bread)	95
Rye (whole meal)	89
Rye (whole grain, i.e. pumpernickel)	68
Wheat (white)	100
Wheat (whole meal)	100
Pasta	
Macaroni (white, boiled 5 min)	64
Spaghetti (brown, boiled 15 min)	61
Spaghetti (white, boiled 15 min)	67
Star pasta (white, boiled 5 min)	54
Cereal Grains	
Barley (pearled)	36
Buckwheat	78
Bulgur	65
Millet	103
Rice (brown)	81
Rice (instant, boiled 1 min)	65
Rice (parboiled, boiled 5 min)	54
Rice (parboiled, boiled 15 min)	68
Rice (polished, boiled 5 min)	58

FOOD	GLYCEMIC INDEX
Cereal Grains (continued)	
Rice (polished, boiled 10–25 min)	81
Rye kernels	47
Sweet corn	80
Wheat kernels	63
Breakfast Cereals	
"All Bran"	74
Cornflakes	121
Muesli	96
Porridge oats	89
Puffed rice	132
Puffed wheat	110
Shredded wheat	97
"Weetebix"	108
Cookies	
Digestive	82
Oatmeal	78
Plain crackers (water biscuits)	100
"Rich Tea"	80
Shortbread cookies	88
Root Vegetables	
Potato (instant)	120
Potato (mashed)	98
Potato (new/white boiled)	80
Potato (Russet, baked)	118
Potato (sweet)	70
Yam	74

FOOD	GLYCEMIC INDEX
Legume	
Baked beans (canned)	70
Bengal gram dal	12
Butter beans	46
Chickpeas (dried)	47
Chickpeas (canned)	60
Frozen Peas	74
Garden peas (frozen)	65
Green peas (canned)	50
Green peas (dried)	65
Haricot beans (white, dried)	54
Kidney beans (dried)	43
Kidney beans (canned)	74
Lentils (green, dried)	36
Lentils (green, canned)	74
Lentils (red, dried)	38
Pinto beans (dried)	80
Pinto beans (canned)	38
Peanuts	15
Soya beans (dried)	20
Soya beans (canned)	22
Fruit	
Apple	52
Apple juice	45
Banana	84

FOOD	GLYCEMIC INDEX
Fruit (continued)	
Grapes	62
Grapefruit	36
Orange	59
Orange juice	71
Peach	40
Pear	47
Plum	34
Raisins	93
Sugars	
Fructose	26
Glucose	138
Honey	126
Lactose	57
Maltose	152
Sucrose	83
Dairy Products	
Custard	59
Ice cream	69
Skim milk	46
Whole milk	44
Yogurt	52
Snack Foods	
Corn chips	99
Potato chips	77

Glycemic Index

The glycemic index is defined as the blood glucose response to a fifty gram available carbohydrate portion of a food expressed as a percentage of the response to the same amount of carbohydrate from a standard food, which has been either glucoside or white bread. In practical terms, this means that each food has the ability to raise blood glucose to variable degrees. The greater the blood glucose level, the greater the insulin response. Thus, we want to choose food with low glycemic indices (see Figure 4). There are many specific benefits of consuming food with low glycemic indices:

- Blood lipids are reduced in hypertriglyceridemic patients.

- Insulin secretion is reduced.

- Overall blood glucose control improves in insulin-dependent and noninsulin-dependent diabetic subjects.

- There is a reduction in abnormal blood glucose, insulin, and amino acid levels in patients with cirrhosis.

- Urinary urea excretion is reduced, presumably by increasing nitrogen trapping by colonic bacteria.

Also, foods with low glycemic indices may enhance satiety, and foods with low glycemic indices may increase athletic performance.

Your body can't produce enough digestive enzymes without the right balance of minerals and B vitamins. Compensating for your sweet tooth with extra healthy foods may be a losing battle since your body is no longer digesting or assimilating food efficiently. *This is another real key for kids and hyperactivity since they are already consuming food that is nutritionally stripped.*

Important Facts:

- Eating sugar puts stress on digestion.

- Poor digestion can lead to allergies.

- Sugar consumption results in poor health.

Sweeteners to Avoid

What about other refined sugars? *Brown sugar* is simply refined sugar that is sprayed with molasses to make it appear more whole. *Turbinado sugar* gives the illusion of health, but is just one step away from white sugar. Tubinado is made from ninety-five percent sucrose (table sugar). It skips only the final filtration stage of sugar refining with little difference in nutritional value. I would say no to Sucralose (Splenda™) and Agave products.

Corn syrup is found everywhere. It is used in everything from bouillon cubes to spaghetti sauce and even in some "natural" juices. Corn syrup processed from cornstarch is almost as sweet as refined sugar and is absorbed quickly by your blood. Corn-derived sweeteners pose other problems: They often contain high levels of pesticide residues that are genetically modified and are common allergy producers. This is a cheap and plentiful sweetener often used in soft drinks, candy, and baked goods. Corn syrup is very similar to refined sugar in composition as well as negative effect.

Aspartame, which is a common synthetic sweetener, affects the nervous system and brain in a very negative way. Aspartame is made from two proteins, or amino acids, which gives it super-sweetness. Aspartame has many harmful effects: behavior changes in children, headaches, dizziness, epileptic-like seizures, and bulging of the eyes to name a few. Aspartame is an "excitotoxin," a substance that over stimulates neurons and causes them to die suddenly (as though they were excited to death). One of the last steps of aspartame metabolism is formaldehyde. The next time you consume diet soda, think. You are literally embalming yourself.

Sucrose is found in white sugar and maple syrup. Sucrose requires very little digestion and provides instant energy followed by plummeting blood sugar levels. It stresses the entire body system.

Glucose is also called dextrose. When combined with sucrose, glucose subjects your blood sugar to the same ups and downs. In whole food form—in starches like beans and whole-grain breads, which are also rich in soluble fiber—glucose takes longer to digest, resulting in more balanced energy.

Sorbitol, Mannitol, and *Zylitol* are synthetic sugar alcohols. Although these can cause less of an insulin jump in glucose than sugar, many people suffer gastric distress. Watch for these listed as ingredients in foods.

Unrefined cane juice. This is sugarcane in crystal form. Nothing more, nothing less. Unrefined cane juice is brown and granulated, contains 85–96.5 percent sucrose, and retains all of sugarcane's vitamins, minerals, and other nutrients. Cane juice has a slightly stronger flavor and less intense sweetness than white sugar. Look for the brand names Sucanat® and Florida Crystals®.

Crystalline fructose. This refined simple sugar has the same molecular structure as fruit sugar. It's almost twice as sweet as white sugar, yet releases glucose into the bloodstream much more slowly. Extra sugar gets stored in your liver as glycogen instead of continuing to flood your bloodstream. Thus, crystalline fructose appeals to diabetics and hypoglycemics.

Sweeteners—The Best of the Naturals

Become sugar-savvy! The term *natural,* as applied to sweeteners, can mean many things. The following recommended sweeteners will provide you with steady energy because they take a long time to digest. Natural choices offer rich flavors, vitamins, and minerals without the ups and downs of refined sugars.

Sugar substitutes were actually the natural sweeteners of days past, especially honey and maple syrup. Stay away from human-made artificial sweeteners including aspartame and any of the "sugar alcohols" (names ending in "ol"). In health food stores, be alert for sugars disguised as "evaporated cane juice" or "cane juice crystals." These can still cause problems, regardless of what the health food store manager tells you. My patients have seen huge improvements by changing their sugar choices.

Brown rice syrup. Your bloodstream absorbs this balanced syrup, high in maltose and complex carbohydrates, slowly and steadily. Brown rice syrup is a natural for baked goods and hot drinks: it adds subtle sweetness and a rich, butterscotch-like flavor. To get sweetness from starchy brown rice, the magic ingredients are enzymes, but the actual process varies depending on the syrup manufacturer. "Malted" syrups use whole sprouted barley to create a balanced sweetener. Choose these syrups to make tastier muffins and cakes. Cheaper, sweeter rice syrups use isolated enzymes and are a bit harder on blood sugar levels. For a healthy treat, drizzle gently heated rice syrup over popcorn to make natural caramel corn! Store in a cool, dry place.

Devansoy™ is the brand name for powdered brown rice sweetener, which contains the same complex carbohydrates as brown rice syrup as well as a natural plant flavoring.

Barley malt syrup. This sweetener is made much like rice syrup, but it uses sprouted barley to turn grain starches into a complex sweetener that is digested slowly. Use barley malt syrup to add molasses-like flavor and light sweetness to beans, cookies, muffins, and cakes. Store in cool, dry place.

Amasake is an ancient, Oriental whole-grain sweetener made from cultured brown rice. It has a thick, pudding-like consistency. Baked goods benefit from amasake's subtle sweetness, moisture, and leavening power.

Stevia is a sweet South American herb that has been safely used by many cultures for centuries. Extensive scientific studies confirm these ancient claims to safety. However, the FDA has approved it only when labeled as a dietary supplement, not as a sweetener. Advocates consider stevia to be one of the healthiest sweeteners as well as a tonic for healing skin. Stevia is 150 to 400 times sweeter than white sugar, has no calories, and can actually regulate blood sugar levels. Unrefined stevia has a molasses-like flavor; refined stevia (popular in Japan) has less flavor and nutrients.

Fruitsource®. This brand-name sweetener combines the sweetness of grape juice concentrate with the complex carbohydrates of brown rice syrup. *FruitSource* is light

177

amber in color and eighty percent as sweet as white sugar. Look for *FruitSource* in liquid and granulated form. *Liquid Plus*, a similar product, better matches the sweetness of white sugar. Whichever form you choose, the options are better for your blood sugar than refined sugar!

Whole fruit. For baking, try fruit purees, dried fruit, and cooked fruit sauces or butters. The less water remaining in a fruit, the more concentrated its flavor and sugar content. You'll find fiber and naturally balanced nutrients in whole fruits like apples, bananas, and apricots. To add mild sweetness and moisture to baked goods, mix in the magic of mashed winter squashes, sweet potatoes, and carrots!

Fructose: A very sweet sugar found in fruits and honey and used as a food preservative and an intravenous nutrient. Fructose in whole foods provides balanced energy.

Honey. It takes one bee an entire lifetime to produce a single tablespoon of honey from flower nectar. But that small amount goes a long way! Honey is mostly made of glucose and fructose and is up to twice as sweet as white sugar. Honey enters the bloodstream rapidly. Buy raw honey, which still contains some vitamins, minerals, enzymes, and pollen. Honeys vary in color (according to their flower source) and range in strength from mild clover to strong orange blossom. A benefit of eating honey produced in your geographical region is that it may reduce hay fever and allergy symptoms by bolstering your natural immunity. Note: raw honey can lead to a toxic, even fatal form of botulism in children under one year of age. Limit honey consumption; it does result in similar results as sucrose.

Maltose is the primary sugar in brown rice and barley malt syrups. Maltose is a complex sugar that is digested slowly. It is the sugar with "staying power."

Maple syrup. It takes about ten gallons of maple sap to produce one gallon of maple syrup. Like honey, a little goes a long way. Maple syrup is roughly sixty-five percent sucrose and contains small amounts of trace minerals. Maple syrup has a rich taste and is absorbed fairly quickly into the bloodstream. Select real maple syrup that has no added corn syrup. Also, look for syrups that come from organic producers who don't use formaldehyde to prolong sap flow. Grade A syrups come from the first tapping: they range in color from light to dark amber. Grade B syrups come from the last tapping; they have more minerals and a stronger flavor and color.

Date sugar. This sweetener is made from dried, ground dates, is light brown, and has a sugary texture. Date sugar retains many naturally occurring vitamins and minerals, is sixty-five percent sucrose, and has a fairly rapid effect on blood sugar. Use it in baking in place of brown sugar, but reduce your baking time or temperature in order to prevent premature browning. Store in a cool, dry place.

Concentrated fruit juice. All concentrates are not created equally. Highly refined juice sweeteners are labeled "modified." These sweeteners, similar to white sugar, have lost both their fruit flavor and their nutrients. Better choices are fruit concentrates that have been evaporated in a vacuum. These retain rich fruit flavors and aromas along with many vitamins and minerals. Carefully read labels on cereal, cookie, jelly, and beverage containers, then choose products with the highest percentage of real fruit juice. Beware of white grape juice concentrates that aren't organic; their pesticide residues can be high!

Blackstrap molasses. Molasses, a by-product of sugar production, is a highly-processed simple sugar that enters the bloodstream rapidly. Molasses may also contain chemical residues associated with the growing and refining of white sugar. If you grew up on conventional molasses, your taste buds may have to adjust to the softer bite of blackstrap molasses, which contains high amounts of balancing minerals such as calcium, iron, potassium, magnesium, zinc, copper, and chromium. Use it as a sweetener in cakes, pies, and cookies. Barbados molasses is sweeter and more syrupy than blackstrap; it is perfect for baking, but lacks blackstrap's minerals. (Note: *Diabetics should not use any type of molasses.*)

Sugar Substitution

Note: Amount indicates the equivalent of one cup of white sugar.

Sweetener	Amount	Liquid Reduction	Suggested Use
Honey	½–⅔ cup	¼ cup	All-purpose
Maple syrup	½–¾ cup	¼ cup	Baking and Desserts
Maple sugar	½–⅓ cup	None	Baking and Candies
Barley malt syrup	1–1½ cups	½ cup	Breads and Baking
Rice syrup	1–1⅓ cups	½ cup	Baking and Cakes
Date sugar	⅔ cup	None	Breads and Baking
Blackstrap Molasses	½ cup	¼ cup	Breads and Baking
Fruit juice concentrate	1 cup	⅓ cup	All-purpose
Stevia	1 tsp/cup of water	1 cup	Baking

(Note: If you have a serious blood sugar regulation problem, such as diabetes or hypoglycemia, see your healthcare practitioner to determine the type and amount of sweeteners your body can handle.)

Day 127

Grapes of Wrath

Woe is me! For I am like those who gather summer fruits,
like those who glean vintage grapes... (Micah 7:1).

The fruit of the vine is grapes. Jesus' first miracle while on earth involved the natural by-product of grapes—wine. Grapes, wine, and vines are referenced often throughout the Bible.

Patients who have an issue with blood sugar fluctuations, commonly called hypoglycemia, appear to be more sensitive to sweet fruits. Are you one of those unsuspecting individuals? Here's a question for you. Do you crave bananas, raisins, dried fruit, dates, figs, or grapes?

Patients often come into my office with fatigue and pain. Ask yourself if your left neck hurts on a regular basis If so, go to your food journal and look at some of the items I mentioned. They may be your problem. Eliminate them from your diet and focus on greens and protein. For one month, slowly incorporate pears, plums, and one half of an apple back into your diet. I see *huge* whole body restoration and health by eliminating sweet fruits. Yes, you can eat them again, but only in limited rationed amounts.

Natural Prescription for Health: Focus on eating veggies for a sweet fruit replacement.

Personal Thoughts/Goals:

_____

_____

_____

_____

Day 128

The Prodigal Son

*And he would gladly have fed on and filled his belly with carob pods
that the hogs were eating...* (Luke 15:16 AMP).

The prodigal son was feeding pigs carob pods—while he was starving to death. Carob is used frequently as a chocolate substitute (not a sugar alternative). It is mixed with saturated fats and sugar or sugar substitute during processing. Some carob bars actually contain more saturated fat than chocolate bars.

Carob is a possible replacement for people with chocolate allergies. Carob does have a fair amount of protein as well as some calcium and phosphorous, and it does have B vitamins and minerals. Carob is available in tablet, powder, syrup, and wafer forms. Make sure you read labels and look at the source of sweeteners in the products with carob. Don't be fooled. Evaporated cane juice or crystals is still sugar. Carob serves as an excellent illustration that excessive use of any "natural" substance can have its own health risks.

Natural Prescription for Health: Carob chips are an option for milk chocolate. Read labels, avoid sugar.

Personal Thoughts/Goals:

_____

_____

_____

_____

Day 129

Honey—A Sweet Alternative

My son, eat honey because it is good, and the honeycomb
which is sweet to your taste (Proverbs 24:13).

One of the God-designed sweets is honey. It is mentioned over fifty times in the Bible. Honey is obviously a sweetener designed as a food. What you might not know about honey is that if you eat too much, you may vomit. *"Eat only as much as you need..."* (Prov. 25:16). Honey is controversial in that some feel it has the same effect on diet as sugar while others say it does not produce the same results.

Honey is not refined sugar. My experience reveals that patients do not appear to get addicted to honey like they do refined sugar. However, honey does cause left neck pain. The pancreas must do some type of extra work to process it. Natural honey from a local beekeeper promotes health. Honey has over 150 ingredients, such as collagen with a protein called proline. My suggestion is to slowly divert your sugar cravings to honey.

Natural Prescription for Health: Plan to take a drive in your area to find and secure a local source of honey from a beekeeper. Ask for a source at your local health food store.

Personal Thoughts/Goals:

_____

_____

_____

_____

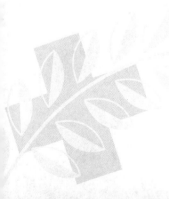

Day 130

Spiritual Arm Wrestling

All things are lawful for me, but all things are not helpful. All things are lawful for me, but I will not be brought under the power of any. (1 Corinthians 6:12)

Our bodies are the temple of the Holy Spirit who, if we have asked Jesus into our hearts, is living in us. We are not our own for we were bought at a price. Therefore, we must glorify God in our bodies and in our spirits.

Whether in the office, while speaking to groups, or during televised programs, I fondly tell listeners that sugar is from the devil. Sugar paralyzes the immune system, thus promoting death. Satan came to steal, kill, and destroy, and I believe sugar has the potential to sabotage our walk with the Lord.

Natural Prescription for Health: Add whole food chromium to your supplement routine if you crave sugar.

Personal Thoughts/Goals:

_____

_____

_____

_____

Day 131

Life Is in the Sap

The trees of the Lord are full of sap... (Psalm 104:16).

Our Heavenly Father thought about our every need. Imagine the delight on the taste buds of the first person who sampled the initial batch of boiled sap.

Maple syrup from the tree (without high fructose corn syrup added to it, as in commercial products) is a viable alternative to refined, white crystalline sugar. It takes about ten gallons of maple sap to produce one gallon of maple syrup. Like honey, a little goes a long way. Maple syrup is approximately sixty-five percent sucrose (table sugar) and contains small amounts of trace minerals. Real maple syrup has a rich taste and is absorbed fairly quickly into the bloodstream. Select real maple syrup that has *no added high fructose corn syrup.* Also look for syrups that come from organic producers who don't use formaldehyde to prolong sap flow. Grade A syrups come from the first tapping. They range in color from light to dark amber. Grade B syrups come from the last tapping. They have more minerals and a stronger flavor and color.

Natural Prescription for Health: Use maple syrup as an alternative to sugar. One fourth cup of maple syrup is equivalent to one half cup of sugar (see Glycemic Foods chart, pages 171–174).

Personal Thoughts/Goals:

_____

_____

_____

_____

Day 132

The Sugar/Fat Connection

The Lord said to me, "What do you see, Jeremiah" and I said, "Figs, the good figs... and the bad, very bad, which cannot be eaten..." (Jeremiah 24:3).

Fruit has been with humankind since creation. God created food for our pleasure and necessity, yet eating an excess of any one item over time can create an imbalance and dysfunction, even fruit.

I know we have been told to eat our five servings of fruit and vegetables daily. I wholeheartedly agree that we need to eat that amount to be at a minimum. My experience reveals that many people focus on the sweet and super-sweet dried fruits, resulting in a carbohydrate overdose. Your body requires a limited amount of all of the primary building blocks: carbohydrates, fats, and proteins. When you focus on and consume the sweeter fruits or carbs, your body will convert them to fat. This might not be a habit of yours, but I have seen patients eat their "normal" cake, cookie, doughnut, and Danish then add fruit to the mix and think that it doesn't count. Hello?! *All* food is accounted for. Excess fruit can be converted to *fat!* And fat needs to be used or burned.

Natural Prescription for Health: Limit sweet fruits like bananas, raisins, and grapes. Avoid or limit *all* dried fruit, including apricots, prunes, dates, and figs.

Personal Thoughts/Goals:

_____

_____

_____

_____

Day 133

Fit Versus Fat

You're better off fit and fat than just fat, but fitness doesn't counter all the risk of excess flab.

In a study that tracked more than 116,000 women for twenty-four years, those who were active and weren't overweight had the lowest risk of dying sooner than expected. (*Active* meant that the women did at least three-and-a-half hours a week of moderate-to-vigorous exercise like brisk walking.) Compared to those women, the risk was:

- Twenty-eight percent higher for active women who were overweight

- Fifty-five percent higher for inactive women (they did less than one hour of exercise a week) who were not overweight

- Sixty-four percent higher for inactive women who were overweight

Even a modest weight gain (about ten to twenty pounds) after age eighteen raised the risk of premature death by fifteen percent. Among women who never smoked, excess weight and inactivity accounted for an estimated fifty-nine percent of deaths from heart attack or stroke and twenty-one percent of deaths from cancer.

Natural Prescription for Health: Keep moving. And try to lose excess weight.

Before making Dr. DeMaria's recommended lifestyle changes, I had stomach issues, mid-back tightness, lower back discomfort after physical activity, and neck soreness when turning to the side. I modified my eating habits by eliminating milk and cheese and cutting down on processed foods. The education on food ingredients has helped tremendously with shopping and planning meals for me and my family. The concept provided by Dr. DeMaria's office of good nutrition and exercise is what I believe is the future of all-around wellness. —Lori Kotanidee

Personal Thoughts/Goals:

_____

_____

_____

_____

Day 134

Feed Your Humpty Dumpty Body Right

It is sown a natural body, it is raised a spiritual body.
There is a natural body and there is a spiritual body (1 Corinthians 15:44).

There is much confusion today in the area of ideal weight levels. The variety of body types and circumstances, including childbirth and discipline to control appetite, need to be considered. The body's energy system works very effectively with carbohydrate consumption. Fruits and vegetables burn very well in a clean machine. A stressed pancreas from refined sugar, low thyroid function antagonized by chlorine, and an overworked adrenal gland fuel pump from too many activities and personal stress, creates an imbalance resulting in more refined sugar cravings.

Refined food depletes cortisol, a hormone from the adrenals, which is required to shut off insulin when protein in the diet is low. When insulin stays elevated, your extra carbs are converted to fat around the belly in males and buttocks in females. Over time, with a breakdown of adrenal and pancreas function, exhaustion occurs. Once exhausted, the body no longer burns carbs effectively and, therefore, cannot provide fuel for the body. At that point, your body begins to rob muscle of nutrients. Arms begin to break down, first resulting in skinny arms and legs. You end up with a "Humpty Dumpty" physique. It is best to then minimize refined carbs and sweet fruits and focus on more protein. Build up your natural body to maintain an A-1 spiritual body.

Natural Prescription for Health: Avoid high glycemic foods (see Glycemic Foods chart, pages 171–174).

Personal Thoughts/Goals:

_____

_____

_____

_____

Day 135

Say No to Sugar Substitutes

*Also take for yourself quality spices—five hundred shekels of liquid myrrh,
half as much sweet-smelling cinnamon…two hundred and fifty
shekels of sweet-smelling cane…* (Exodus 30:23).

I prefer natural complex sugars such as brown rice syrup, pear sweet, maltose, pure maple syrup, honey, and even organic evaporated cane juice (very small amounts of the cane juice) versus any human-made substitute. Every few years a newer, safer, human-made sugar alternative promises to be sweet and safe. Nothing made by people will ever be safe enough for people to consume. All the commercial brands eventually create a negative toxic situation including damage to the liver, which processes and filters all chemicals.

Aspartame, like other fake sweeteners, appears to be created by innocent ingredients, *but* the final product can be totally different in character from what the body is able to tolerate and use. Unhealthy cravings for sweets are signs of a deep-rooted problem such as yeast overgrowth and mineral deficiencies. Aspartame can affect vision and can cause headaches, rashes, and even seizures. The excitotoxins in aspartame affect brain function. Diet soda drinkers beware that some of your health issues can be related to the sweetener source.

Natural Prescription for Health: Increase chromium supplement intake if you crave sweets. Switch to grape juice spritzers as an alternative to sugary corn syrup soda.

Personal Thoughts/Goals:

_____

_____

_____

_____

Day 136

The Devil's Candy

You shall eat and not be satisfied; hunger shall be in your midst... (Micah 6:14).

Are you hungry? A typical question posed by the fast food industry to lure you in for a meal. Satan came to steal, kill, and destroy. He lurks everywhere—mammon or money is often his bait.

The human body uses various forms of glucose or carbohydrates as fuel. When you eat certain whole foods versus processed or human-made foods, your body will respond with insulin. Insulin is used by the body to get fuel or glucose into the cells.

There is another transmitter released that tells your brain that you have consumed fuel and that you are full or finished. Your appetite is turned off. The food manufacturers have found an inexpensive sweetener that bypasses the insulin step so you can eat and eat and still be hungry. The sweetener is called high fructose corn syrup. Do not be fooled by the word fructose—it's safe in whole foods, but alone as *high fructose corn syrup* it can lead to obesity. Read food product labels.

Natural Prescription for Health: *Red Alert*: High fructose corn syrup is detrimental to your health. HFCS can deplete leptin, which is a hormone used by the body to signal you are full. Eating foods with HFCS, even applesauce or a beverage, may be the reason you are always hungry. Leptin levels can be assessed using noninvasive galvanic skin response bio-communication technology.

Personal Thoughts/Goals:

_____

_____

_____

_____

Day 137

Side Pain

*And the Lord God caused a deep sleep to fall on Adam, and he slept; and He took one of his **ribs**, and closed up the flesh in its place. Then the **rib** which the Lord God had taken from man He made into a woman… (Genesis 2:21-22, emphasis added).*

Did you ever have severe, intense pain that is worse when breathing, often on the left side, the kind of pain that imitates a heart attack?

Adam contributed a rib for the creation of Eve. Ribs can move and can come out of alignment or become "subluxated." Ribs have an attachment to vertebrae in the mid-back or thoracic spine. There are several other possibilities eliciting pain in the rib region, including kidney stones, ulcers, shingles, lung irritation, and referral from internal organs.

Forward postural alignment with round shoulders is a sign of weakness of the supporting trunk structures. I have found raking leaves with the twisting movement creates enormous pressure on the ribs and small muscles in between them. Besides an injury or trauma, I also know that what you eat, especially sweet foods and drinks, can weaken supporting structures, possibly resulting in the displacement of a rib, causing relentless pain.

Natural Prescription for Health: Avoid sugar, bananas, raisins, and grapes that could cause rib pain.

Personal Thoughts/Goals:

_____

_____

_____

_____

Day 138

"I Scream, You Scream, We All Scream for Ice Cream!"

He asked for water, she gave milk; she brought out cream in a lordly bowl (Judges 5:25).

"*My son, eat honey because it is good, and the honeycomb which is sweet to your taste*" (Prov. 24:13). Let's be real. We all like sweet foods. The challenge is to not let the sweets have us. Sugar-loaded alcohol enslaves people in a devastating yoke. Ice cream can create an addiction, resulting in unsuspecting symptoms including sinusitis, headaches, pancreas stress, acne, and colon issues.

I have assessed and treated pancreas cancer successfully. After a thorough evaluation of the patient's diet history, I was able to determine that the pancreatic cancer was possibly linked to regular ice cream consumption. Why? Be mindful of the additives used to flavor ice cream. Some of the artificial flavors are potent poisons powerful enough to cause liver, kidney, pancreas, and heart damage. Benzyl acetate is a synthetic chemical that imparts a strawberry flavor. Ethyl acetate is used by many manufacturers to give ice cream a pineapple flavor; it is also used as a leather cleanser. Peperonal is used in place of vanilla and is also used to kill lice. Vanillin, used as a vanilla flavor, is from wood pulp. Amyl butgrate is used to replace banana and is also a paint solvent.

Natural Prescription for Health: Whole cream without additives or chemical enhancers is the logical choice. Read ingredient labels.

Personal Thoughts/Goals:

_____

_____

_____

_____

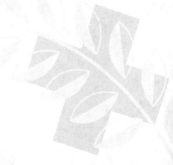

Day 139

Elijah's Cake

…Go and do as you have said, but make me a small cake from it first, and bring it to me; and afterward make some for yourself and your son (1 Kings 17:13).

How would you like someone to take your very last morsel of food? The widow responded to the request and created a small flour cake for Elijah to eat. She literally created the first documented pastry business with her cake or doughnut.

Today's doughnut is hardly the same cake Elijah ate. The modern, deep-fried doughnut should be called Do-Nots. Let's have a little doughnut talk. The average doughnut adds a minimum of three hundred calories. The trans fat alone will do enough damage to your cell membranes and nervous system to cripple your body's ability to communicate for up to 102 days (the double half-life of trans fat). The several teaspoons of sugar stop your white blood cells from fulfilling the responsibility in their job description, which is to seek and destroy bacteria, viruses, free radicals, and cancer. Wheat is a common allergen creating digestive distress. The cream filling and frosting has enough arachidonic acid-producing prostaglandin #2 to cause pain in every joint in your body. Elijah never had to worry about that. I tell my patients that doughnuts are like lethal smart bombs.

Natural Prescription for Health: Replace breakfast Do-Nots with quinoa, a gluten-free oatmeal replacement, or short grain brown rice with almonds and applesauce and cinnamon.

Personal Thoughts/Goals:

_____

_____

_____

_____

Day 140

Does Timing Matter?

Thanks to hectic schedules, many people no longer eat breakfast, lunch, and dinner at the same time every day. And that may be fueling the bulging American waistline.

Obese women who were told to eat six meals a day on a regular schedule burned more calories after meals than when they were instructed to eat anywhere from three to nine meals a day on an irregular schedule. (They were told to eat seven meals the first day, four the next, then nine, three, and so forth.)

The women also had lower LDL ("bad") cholesterol and lower peak insulin levels on the regular meal schedule. An earlier study found similar results in lean women. This study isn't conclusive because each eating routine lasted just two weeks (which may explain why weight didn't change in either group).[24]

Natural Prescription for Health: The study does suggest, though, that snacking, meals on the run, and a chaotic eating schedule may make it harder to stay lean.

> I used to always get sick and had to miss work due to bronchitis. I had pain in my lungs and overall weakness from this condition. I regularly took over-the-counter cough syrup and pain pills. Following Dr. DeMaria's advice, I started eating more fruits and vegetables and began drinking more water. I have cut out most of the white sugar in my diet.

> The information and care provided by Dr. Bob has turned my life around. I feel like a new person. I am so thankful that I had friends that referred me to him. My bronchitis attacks have ceased. I miss very little work now due to better health. I have not had a cold since I started drugless healthcare one and a half years ago. All of my family members are now treated by Dr. Bob, and they have also enjoyed better health after their care. —Betty White

Personal Thoughts/Goals:

_____

_____

_____

_____

Day 141

Stevia—Sweetener

...Take and eat it and it [synthetic sweeteners]*; will make your stomach bitter, but it will be as sweet as honey in your mouth* (Revelation 10:9).

Sugar is a secret killer in America. Sugar is lurking in packaged entrees, condiments, sauces, dressings, and soups. It can be found in nearly every imaginable commercially available item in conventional grocery stores. Tip: Always make a shopping list and never shop when you are hungry. Read labels as though you were on a reconnaissance mission—like a trained soldier. Eat as a cave man would—whole food, grains, veggies, and fruit.

Not recognized as a sweetener by the US government, stevia, a South American herb, is two hundred to three hundred times sweeter than regular sugar. Stevia has no calories, is suitable for diabetics, does not cause cavities, and is heat stable, which means it can be used for cooking and baking. Stevia is a great alternative to synthetic sweeteners. It blends easily with honey, and it has been safely consumed in many countries around the world for decades.

Stevia grows about eighteen inches tall with small, narrow leaves. I pluck stevia leaves from the top down and dry them in a piloted oven or dehydrator then store the dried leaves in an air tight container. The leaves are then easily powdered in a blender. Sprinkle the green herb on any item you generally sweeten with sugar or substitute.

Natural Prescription for Health: Splenda is chlorinated sucrose derivatives. It enlarges the liver and kidneys and shrinks the thymus. Plant some stevia in your garden!

Personal Thoughts/Goals:

_____

_____

_____

_____

Day 142

How Sweet Is Sweet Enough?

The thief [satan-sugar] *does not come except to steal* [nutrients],
and to kill, and destroy... (John 10:10).

Satan came to steal, kill, and destroy. By far, in my experience of treating the most serious conditions, sugar seems to always be at the pivotal starting point. Watch what you feed your kids. Brightly colored packaged treats found at the movie theater and convenience stores should raise a suspicious eye. One particular "movie candy" that I recently evaluated had sugar, high fructose corn syrup, hydrogenated fat, and multiple toxic dyes. After eating this "treat," unsuspecting kids instantly have brain waves that misfire, possibly creating behavioral issues.

I have discovered that sport drinks and power bars commonly found in athletic facilities, conventional grocery stores, and health food stores are stealthy candy bars. Be aware of "evaporated organic cane juice crystals," which is sugar in disguise. I avoid *all* human-made synthetic sugars. Manitol, sorbitol, and xylitol are alcohol-based sweeteners marketed as "sugar free" which create additional stress to the detox system. Seek grape juice sweetened, brown rice syrup, stevia, honey or pear sweet as natural-sourced sweeteners.

Natural Prescription for Health: Read labels; do not be fooled by organic evaporated cane crystals.

Personal Thoughts/Goals:

_____

_____

_____

_____

Day 143

Pass the Honey

*Have you found honey? Eat only as much as you need lest
you be filled with it and vomit* (Proverbs 25:16).

Honey is talked about throughout the Bible. Honey can be an excellent source of a natural sweetener, *but* I have seen major issues with overdoing honey similar to what I see with sugar consumption. Honey is ninety-five percent sucrose, and sucrose is sugar. Yes, honey is not white table sugar, but I have treated patients with chronic pain who use honey as a sugar substitute and suffer with sugar headaches, pain syndromes, mood swings, depression, and so forth just like those who consume sugar.

Through my clinical experience, I have been able to correlate pain in the body with consuming sweets. The pain is because most Americans have pancreas and liver burnout which are the two organs, along with others, necessary for proper sugar metabolism. Because of sugar abuse, they no longer properly metabolize sugar, resulting in pain.

I do not encourage the use of honey that is commercially prepared. Consume honey from your geographic region, but go easy on it. Do not use it every day. In fact, try going without sweets for a few weeks. You will feel better!

Natural Prescription for Health: Only consume non-processed honey that is gathered by honey bees from *your* region.

Personal Thoughts/Goals:

_____

_____

_____

_____

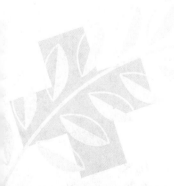

Day 144

The Armor of God

*Put on the whole armor of God, that you may be able
to stand against the wiles of the devil* (Ephesians 6:11).

God knows we need to be protected in the spirit realm. Paul discusses putting on the whole armor of God to protect us from the invisible attacks, of which we may not even be aware.

Your immune system is working 24/7. A properly functioning digestive system is critical for immune function. The colon is one area where fighter cells originate and water is needed to keep the lymph system flowing freely of toxin residues. In the liver, a group of cells called kupffer cells neutralize unwanted bacteria, viruses, parasites, and even cancer cells. Mobilization of the upper mid-back vertebrae increases the capacity of certain immune cells called P.M.N. Sugar, when you eat it, paralyzes the immune system for hours. One white blood cell (WBC) can handle fourteen bacteria in half an hour. Consuming a soda handcuffs the WBC so it can only handle ten, and eating a brownie reduces WBC activity to five. Enjoying Grandma's apple pie or a banana split sabotages the WBC to handle only one bacterium. My suggestion is to polish your armor with healthy food. Sugar tarnishes your protective covering.

Natural Prescription for Health: Mini-trampoline jumping and/or any activity facilitates immune system activity.

Personal Thoughts/Goals:

_____

_____

_____

_____

Day 145

Label Readers

…When it is evening you say, "It will be fair weather, for the sky is red"; and in the morning, "It will be foul weather today, for the sky is red…" (Matthew 16:2).

Red night, sailors delight; red morning, sailor warning. Jesus also spoke of what to look for when the endtime draws near. We stop, look, and listen before crossing the street. Therefore, we read the ingredient labels on the food we eat. The public is more aware that what they eat affects their health.

Much has happened in the food world in just the last few years. At one point, health conscious manufacturers used brown rice syrup, honey, maltose, or barley malt as sweeteners. But many of these companies, with excellent reputations and quality products, were purchased by conventional, profit-driven large food conglomerates. The bottom line: processed, human-made ingredients cost less.

Buyer beware! When you go into a health food store or health food department in a large conventional chain, read the ingredients on the label. Evaporated, organic cane juice is still *sugar*. Raw, organic cane crystals are *sugar*. Do not be duped. Write a letter or voice your opinion to these companies or the store that has them on their shelves.

Natural Prescription for Health: Read the label on your "healthy" power bar. It may contain hidden sugar sources.

Personal Thoughts/Goals:

_____

_____

_____

_____

Day 146

Knowledge Is Power

My people are destroyed for lack of knowledge... (Hosea 4:6).

I was with a friend who dumped two bags of "raw sugar" into her coffee. I could not believe her addiction was so intense. She was surprised to learn that raw sugar was the same as table sugar.

Let me tell you something straight. Jesus came to give us life and give it to the fullest abundance. Satan came to steal, kill, and destroy. Sugar is from the devil. Raw sugar, sometimes called turbinado, is only one refining step away from table sugar or sucrose.

Sugar handcuffs your white blood cells from performing their job. A can of soda with nine-and-a-half teaspoons of sugar can depress your immune system by up to twenty-five percent for five to six hours. And that is just one can! People who eat sugar are always sick and never one hundred percent healthy.

Natural Prescription for Health: Stevia, honey, or maple syrup are alternative sweeteners to sugar.

Personal Thoughts/Goals:

_____

_____

_____

_____

Day 147

Stones and Pounds

How many extra pounds increase your odds of getting a kidney stone? The risk is significantly higher in men who gain about eleven pounds and in women who gain about twenty-five pounds after age twenty (compared to those who gain no weight).

The risk also rises if your waist measures at least thirty-seven inches (men or younger women) or at least thirty-one inches (older women). The risk increases more as you add more pounds or inches.[25]

Natural Prescription for Health: Lose excess weight, but not too quickly. Rapid weight loss can increase the risk of kidney stones.

> I had a kidney stone infection when I came to see Dr. DeMaria. He told me to take a lemon, cut in into four pieces, and put it in hot water with parsley. Then eat the lemon and drink the water. I followed his advice exactly, and it really did help me. I could go to the bathroom and it didn't hurt as badly. It used to be that I could not do all my dishes without occasionally stopping. Now I feel stronger and I can do them. Everyone tells me how much better I look. I think so, too! I really like his seminars and enjoy them. He really helps and makes you better. He is a very good doctor. —Lottie Ward

Personal Thoughts/Goals:

_____

_____

_____

_____

Self-Assessment
Snack Debriefing

Answer the following questions and score accordingly. Your goal is a score of five.

_____ Do you eat mini meals and mid-glycemic index snacks? Add one.

_____ Do you eat sweet or dried fruits (bananas, raisins, grapes) throughout the day? Subtract one.

_____ Do you eat raw almonds or walnuts during the day? Add one.

_____ Do you drink unsweetened drinks? Add one.

_____ Do you eat candy bars or sugar-sweetened "protein" energy bars? Subtract one.

_____ Do you have a pastry, Danish, or doughnut as a midmeal snack? Subtract one.

_____ Are fresh cut veggies in your daily food plan? Add one.

_____ Do soda, novelty coffee drinks, or commercial juices satisfy your "hunger pains"? Subtract one.

_____ Do you start your day with a measured amount of pure water? Add one.

_____ Do you eat several small meals daily? Add one.

_____ Do you eat right before bed? Subtract one.

_____ Do you eat peanuts, pizza, snack cakes? Subtract one.

_____ Do you eat snacks with trans fat? Subtract one.

_____ Do you eat non-wheat snacks? Add one.

_____ Total score

Dr. Bob's snack comment: Continuous "grazing" may keep your blood sugar steady, but also stresses the digestive system. Focus on snacks that do not cause a large insulin release. The Glycemic Index midrange is best (see the introduction to this section). Sweets can be addictive, resulting in extra pounds and an underlying cause of pain.

Digestion—Not Indigestion

Jesus talked about digestion in His parables. You are not only what you eat, but also what you digest and absorb. Poor digestion can result in food that is not broken down to proper size. Food enters and leaves the body. What you decide to eat becomes you. It is serious. Regular daily elimination is essential for optimal well-being. You would do best to eat fresh, organic fiber foods to assist colon elimination.

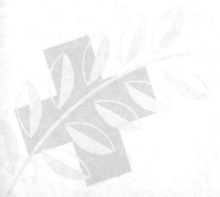

Day 148

Your Liver—Your Lifeline

Till an arrow struck his liver... (Proverbs 7:23).

The liver is an incredible organ with hundreds of known functions. It is so highly regarded in Eastern and Asian cultures that newlyweds figuratively exchange livers instead of the heart as we are accustomed to in Western societies.

The liver is commonly seen as the literal "oil filter" of the body—but it does so much more. Reserves of blood are stored in the liver along with fat soluble vitamins, including A, D, E, and K. Your liver creates bile necessary for proper metabolism of fat. Kupffer cells are active in a healthy liver, seeking and destroying unhealthy invaders, including cancer cells and parasites. Toxins (modern-day arrows) from the air, water, and processed foods and drinks stress the liver.

Natural Prescription for Health: Add Dr. Bob's ABC's to your *daily* routine, one-half of an Apple, a portion of grated raw or baked Beets, and a moderate Carrot for optimal liver function.

Personal Thoughts/Goals:

_____

_____

_____

_____

Day 149

"And Make Bread for Yourself"

Also, take for yourself wheat, barley, lentils, millet and spelt;
put them into one vessel, and make bread of them for yourself (Ezekiel 4:9).

Ezekiel was instructed to make multi-grain bread. Bread and grains are discussed throughout the Bible and have become a foundation in the current US food plate. Be aware that lurking in the plastic wrapper may be ingredients that can negatively affect your health.

Corn syrup, sugar, hydrogenated fats, and colors sabotage normal bodily function. I have encouraged patients with tremors, digestive disturbances, sleep apnea, and pain syndromes to limit wheat bread and see miraculous results. The protein in wheat bread, called gluten, literally glues the villi in your intestine together, diminishing absorption.

Craving bread can be a body signal that you may have a wheat and/or yeast sensitivity. Vary the grains in the bread you use. Try spelt, millet, rice, oat or barley flour bread.

Natural Prescription for Health: Rotate your bread choices to include a sprouted grain variety.

Personal Thoughts/Goals:

_____

_____

_____

_____

Day 150

Daniel's Menu

But Daniel purposed in his heart that he would not defile himself [eat pork] *with the portion of the king's delicacies, nor with the wine which he drank…* (Daniel 1:8).

Daniel was a very wise young man. He had God's favor on his life and the wisdom not to choose items consumed by the kings and royalty. Food consumed in Daniel's day was not refrigerated. Animal flesh that is not cooked or stored properly can result in digestive distress. Sickness would have kept Daniel away from his training and studies. Fruit, vegetables, and grains are generally easily digested and do not create an unhealthy digestive environment.

Daniel, during his fast, while waiting on the Lord to answer his prayer request (see Daniel chapter 10), once again abstained from delicacies involving meat. I wonder if Daniel had blood type A. I have noticed that patients with blood type A have distress with meat products. Do you get distress after eating animal products? Limit the amount of red meat you eat. Focus on eating organic chicken and turkey and a secure source of deep ocean fish. You have to be very aware that fish today is one of the most counterfeited foods. I would not eat farmed fish. Review your diet journal. How do you feel after eating red meat meals?

Natural Prescription for Health: Digestive distress caused by eating meat products, especially for people with blood type A, may require a digestive support with Betaine Hydrochloride—one tablet with each protein meal.

Personal Thoughts/Goals:

_____

_____

_____

_____

Day 151

"Mmmmm Good"

Oh, taste and see that the Lord is good... (Psalm 34:8).

Losing or not having the sense of taste is not fun. I know from experience that when there is congestion in your sinus cavity and you can't taste food, it can make for unpleasant living. You might as well not eat.

My clinical experience suggests that another common cause of not being able to taste is a zinc deficiency. Zinc can be depleted by stress or eating certain grains and protein sources such as wheat and soy. When you have a zinc deficiency, you may notice white spots on your nails, large pores on your face, and excessive scarring at the site of an injury.

Be aware that some fast food companies focus on taste enhancers that can be addictive. The neurons in your brain can be very sensitive to certain chemicals. I have even assessed patients who lost their sense of taste after an automobile accident that damaged neurons.

Natural Prescription for Health: Memory lapses? Avoid zinc-depleting wheat and soy. Snack on fresh, raw pumpkin seeds.

Personal Thoughts/Goals:

_____

_____

_____

_____

Day 152

Bentonite Clay—Toxic Bowel Aide

"O house of Israel, can I not do with you as this potter?" says the Lord. "Look, as the clay is in the potter's hand, so are you in My hand, O house of Israel!" (Jeremiah 18:6).

Jesus is the potter, and we are the clay. Clay, in a skilled potter's hand, can be transformed into magnificent pieces of fine art or containers holding gorgeous bouquets of Hawaiian flowers.

Overdoing it, with too much food, wrong food choices, limited water intake, or excessive toxic exposure can create an intestinal lining on fire. I have a secret weapon for you. It is called Bentonite clay. I use it in my office for patients who have loose stools caused by food poisoning, the flu, or toxic overexposure to a food, drink, or unknown irritant. I do not use it for diagnosed conditions of the colon such as ulcerative colitis.

Bentonite clay is a temporary adsorbent. The toxins attach themselves to the clay. They are not absorbed. The toxins, regardless of the source, are eliminated in bowel movements. I generally suggest one every fifteen minutes until the loose stools cease. This remedy is especially useful for individuals who have an electrolyte level condition, kidney challenges, blood pressure, or diabetes. Always have the physician of your choice monitor your health. The body is self-healing; the clay accelerates the process.

Natural Prescription for Health: Do not eat food that is not totally cooked or tastes spoiled or rotten.

Personal Thoughts/Goals:

_____

_____

_____

_____

Day 153

"Oh, I Ate the Whole Thing!"

Have you found honey? Eat only as much as you need,
lest you be filled with it and vomit (Proverbs 25:16).

Digestive distress is one of the leading reasons why people take medications. I encourage my patients not to drink water or fluids with meals. Fluids dilute or weaken the digestive process and most people do not have enough stomach acid. The diminished acid state, with the presence of fluids, results in poor digestion. You literally can have a compost pile in your stomach, which creates an inorganic acid that people dissolve with antacids, which only compound the problem.

Be aware how you combine foods. I recommend protein with non-starch items. Proteins with greens are a good choice. Protein needs an acid environment. Starches need an alkaline (such as baking soda) environment. I also instruct my patients to eat fruit alone and not to end a meal with it. Eaten with food, the fruit decomposes for hours literally breaking down into alcohol and stressing your system.

Natural Prescription for Health: Do not drink sparkling or "still" water or clear broths with your meals—it dilutes the digestive acid. Drink water *before* and *after*, not during the meal.

Personal Thoughts/Goals:

_____

_____

_____

_____

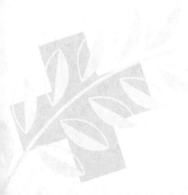

Day 154

Veggies and Diabetes

Yellow-orange and green leafy vegetables may lower the risk of diabetes in overweight women.

Those who averaged one serving of yellow-orange vegetables a day had a twenty-seven percent lower risk of getting diabetes than those who averaged one serving every two weeks. And those who averaged one and a half servings of green leafy vegetables a day had a fourteen percent lower risk than those who averaged one serving a week. The researchers found no link with women who weren't overweight.[26]

Natural Prescription for Health: Though the study needs to be confirmed, it's one more reason to eat nutrient-packed yellow-orange vegetables like carrots, sweet potatoes, and yellow squash and green leafy vegetables like spinach, kale, and lettuce.

> The information received from Dr. DeMaria encourages you make a choice as to what you want to put into your body. When I first came to the office, I had back pain, digestive problems, and some sinus problems. I took Pepto Bismol and Rolaids regularly. I now make conscious decisions reducing my sugar intake and am aware of my general eating habits. I have also greatly reduced my fast food consumption. The most challenging change for me has been to decrease my pop [soda] intake, but after cutting back, the desire is diminishing. —Dean Birdsall

Personal Thoughts/Goals:

_____

_____

_____

_____

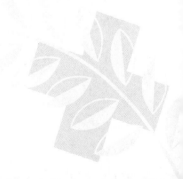

Day 155

Digestion Starts in the Mouth

...Honey and milk are under your tongue... (Song of Solomon 4:11).

The tongue serves so many visual purposes in the Bible. Life and death are in the tongue.

The tongue adds pleasure to eating as your taste buds are located on the tongue. Chew your food long and slowly. The more you chew your food, the better the digestion. Starch digestion requires enzymes that are released by saliva glands in the chewing process. Nutrients are quickly absorbed in the mouth. You might even want to chew your whole food vitamins with the exception of ascorbic acid.

Do you have silver-color, mercury-based, amalgam fillings in your mouth? Mercury is very toxic and interferes with the production of digestive juices released from the parotid glands located in your throat.

I encourage my patients to take chlorophyll capsules and parotid tissue (an animal-based extract) if they have a mouth full of fillings and have allergies. It would be best to have your amalgams removed by a skilled, experienced dentist.

Natural Prescription for Health: Chew your food long and slowly.

Personal Thoughts/Goals:

_____

_____

_____

_____

Day 156

What Is the Glycemic Index?

And they gave him a piece of a cake of figs and two clusters of raisins.
So when he had eaten, his strength came back to him; for he had eaten no bread
nor drank water for three days and nights (1 Samuel 30:12).

When David fed on Egyptian slave's figs and raisins, he was revived. In the New Testament, Saul, prior to being Paul, did not eat for several days before he was filled with the Holy Spirit. The physical person requires fuel just as the spirit person needs to be filled with the Holy Spirit. Acts 9:19 says, *"So when [Saul] had received food, he was strengthened...."*

Our bodies require fuel to flourish. How fast the fuel enters the system can promote or deplete life. The term glycemic index (GI) is simply a ranking of carbohydrates based on their immediate effect on blood glucose (blood sugar levels). Carbohydrates that are slow to break down during digestion have a low GI. Carbohydrates that break down quickly during digestion have a high GI. This state can be likened to throwing gasoline on a fire, resulting in a quick, hot, explosive state—only to quickly cool. These highs and lows tend to stress the status quo. There is a Glycemic Index provided for you in the Glycemic Foods chart on pages 171–174.

You can be on a roller coaster of health with peaks and valleys with headaches, depression, anxiety, pain, dizziness, digestive distress, and more depending on the carbohydrates you choose to eat. A low GI diet results in a smaller rise in blood glucose after meals, which promotes weight loss, helps you stay full longer, and prolongs physical endurance. The fuel you put in your machine affects physical performance.

Natural Prescription for Health: Reduce the amount of white potatoes you eat, especially if you notice the correlation of mid-back pain after eating them. Yams and sweet potatoes do not generally create the same insulin rush.

Personal Thoughts/Goals:

_____

_____

_____

_____

Day 157

Body De-Greaser: Bile

...My bile is poured on the ground... (Lamentations 2:11).

The gallbladder is a reservoir of bile. Bile is produced in the liver. Your liver is a huge factory with functions needed for proper digestion. The liver removes poisonous substances from the blood so they can be expelled from the body. The liver excretes all these gathered toxins as bile. Bile also contains cholesterol and assists the body in processing fats.

Optimal liver function is necessary for bile to flow freely. I encourage my patients to eat at least half an apple daily along with organic beets, either grated raw or baked and diced, not canned or pickled.

Bile can become thick and concentrated forming gallstones. I encourage patients who have had gallbladder surgery to supplement their diet with a bile salt. Eating fiber, apples, and beets facilitates the removal of bile from the body.

Natural Prescription for Health: Eat half an apple daily for fiber and to keep bile flowing freely from the liver.

Personal Thoughts/Goals:

_____

_____

_____

_____

Day 158

Don't Worry—Be Happy

Martha, Martha, you are worried and troubled about many things. But one thing is needed, and Mary has chosen that good part, which will not be taken away from her (Luke 10:41-42).

I am sure that Martha, the sister of Lazarus, was very concerned about the safety of her family friend, Jesus. Do you cry for no reason? Do you have a fear of impending doom, muscle soreness, crave sweets, nervousness, instability, vague fears, depression, anxiety, worry, and apprehension?

These are all common body signals of a little-known but major clinical condition precipitated by lack of whole food B complex. A very common deficiency in Americans today is complex vitamin B. It's not easy to get real B vitamins in the American diet. First of all, the richest source of these vitamins is brewer's yeast (not exactly a staple of the average American). Other sources of B vitamins are whole grains, lamb, nuts, eggs, beans, and brown rice.

Natural Prescription for Health: Do you cry easily or fear impending doom? Add whole food B vitamins to your daily protocol.

Personal Thoughts/Goals:

_____

_____

_____

_____

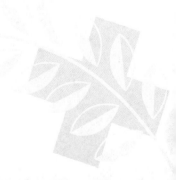

Day 159

Nightshades

*In Him was life, and the life was the light of men. And the **light** shines in the **darkness**, and the darkness did not comprehend it* (John 1:4, emphasis added).

Light is life. God warns us about the activity at night in His Word. There is a classification of food items called *nightshades* that in themselves are not harmful or bad. They have a substance that is a part of their makeup called solanine. Solanine is an irritant to the liver. Your liver needs to be functioning optimally in order for you not to have pain or inflammation caused by the nightshades.

Commonly consumed nightshades include tomatoes, white potatoes, eggplant, and green pepper. In the late summer when tomatoes ripen on the vine and they have that luscious mouthwatering flavor, tasty with basil leaves and olive oil, beware! Eating too many tomatoes with a congested liver can result in intense pain for some. Yet it can be without incident for individuals who are mindful of what they eat. Eating too much of any of the nightshades can create the same state of poor health.

Raw, grated, organic beets or mixed greens promote liver health.

Natural Prescription for Health: Substitute yams and sweet potatoes for white potatoes.

Personal Thoughts/Goals:

_____

_____

_____

_____

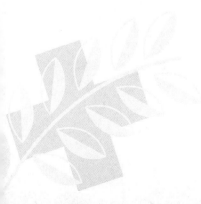

Day 160

Shield Yourself From Perilous Pestilence

Surely he shall deliver you from the snare of the fowler and from the perilous pestilence…. His truth shall be your shield and buckler (Psalm 91:3-4).

The immune system is a shield against invaders. Our bodies are under a tight balance or ecosystem. Tipping the scale can create functional stress and may create toxic overload.

Your lymphatic system does not have a pump like the vascular network. It depends on muscle movement. The lymph system is your sewage and street cleaning department that carries and destroys unfriendly cells, used cells, and organisms. I encourage water consumption and suggest limited dairy, which tends to slow the lymph movement. Your lymphatic network keeps cancer cells in check. Killer lymphocytes, created by your body, act as an invisible shield that protects you.

Cancer growth, which is unchecked cell proliferation, is one of the leading causes of death. To keep this cancer pestilence under control, focus on your body like you do your house. I have my floor drains cleaned. I especially take notice if I smell a foul, stagnant sewer odor. This is an alarm signal that waste water is not leaving the premise. I regularly put eco-friendly pipe cleaner down my sink drain to keep the system working. Keep your system working, too.

Natural Prescription for Health: Halitosis, bad breath, may be a sign of sluggish digestion and poor lymphatic drainage. Combine your foods wisely; reduce liquids with meals.

Personal Thoughts/Goals:

_____

_____

_____

_____

Day 161

Magnesium and Cancer

Magnesium may protect against colorectal cancer, according to a study of more than sixty-one thousand Swedish women.

Those who consumed at least 255 milligrams of magnesium a day (from food and supplements) had about a forty percent lower risk of colorectal cancer than those who consumed less than 209 milligrams a day. Magnesium had protected against colorectal cancer in earlier animal studies.[27]

Natural Prescription for Health: Eat more fruits, vegetables, whole grains, and beans—all of which are rich in magnesium. Multivitamins rarely contain a day's worth—320 milligrams for women and 420 milligrams for men—because the amount needed wouldn't fit into a single tablet.

> When I first came to Dr. Bob, I had spinal pain, I could not sleep at night, and I had a severe case of psoriasis for over twenty-eight years. My elbows use to be sore from the skin problem. I used creams, prescriptions, and over-the-counter remedies, but nothing seemed to help. After receiving spinal subluxation correction care, I feel more energized. After three months of treatment and a change of diet, including taking flax oil, my psoriasis improved, to the point that I am not embarrassed to wear sleeveless tops. My elbows no longer hurt, and the redness and scales have gone away. They are smooth. I teach first graders, which takes a lot of energy, and now I do not feel so tired when I go home. I have more patience with the children in my classroom. I would encourage anyone who reads this to do exactly what Dr. Bob says for your condition. It does work. I am living proof. —Sue Dietz

Personal Thoughts/Goals:

_____

_____

_____

_____

Day 162

The Law of Love

…He who eats, eats to the Lord… (Romans 14:6).

Food is discussed throughout the Bible. In Genesis, food was part of humanity's first confrontation with satan. In Romans chapter 14, Paul is dealing with issues of eating food. Jesus told His disciples that food enters and leaves the body. My research directs me to believe that Jewish people did not eat physically unclean food. People were concerned about what food—*acceptable* to eat by Levitical Law—was being used as an idol offering. Paul did not want a brother to be grieved because of food. Romans 14:15 says, *"…You are no longer walking in love. Do not destroy with your food the one for whom Christ died."* And Romans 14:17 says, *"For the kingdom of God is not eating and drinking, but righteousness and peace and joy in the Holy Spirit."*

Food can be a real issue for some people. I pray that you understand that the concerns I am discussing can physiologically alter your metabolism. Do not get caught up in the "death by denial" trap. Daily in our local paper, I read about individuals who have experienced early death—some are in their thirties and forties. Most, if not all, early deaths can be prevented by eliminating processed food and drinking more water. You should focus on eating meals that include whole grains, organic meat, and vegetables. Determine to eat food that isn't processed.

Natural Prescription for Health: Bake a squash today—add butter, chives, and walnuts.

Personal Thoughts/Goals:

_____

_____

_____

_____

Day 163

Fiber Clean

Jacob gave Esau bread and stew of lentils… (Genesis 25:34).

Fiber-rich food, like beans and legumes, cleanse the small finger-like projecting villi in the digestive system. Fiber helps lower blood cholesterol and stabilizes blood sugar. Beet and oatmeal fiber prevent colon cancer, constipation, hemorrhoids, obesity, and many other disorders. It is also good for removing certain toxic metals from the body. Because the refining process has removed much of the natural fiber from our foods, the typical American diet is lacking fiber. How much fiber is in a fry or jelly doughnut?

Start with small amounts of fiber first, if you have not had any in your diet. Excessive fiber may decrease zinc, iron, and calcium. Always take supplemental fiber separately from other medication or supplements; otherwise, it can lessen their strength and effectiveness.

Make sure your diet contains these high fiber foods: whole-grain cereals and flour, brown rice, nuts, flax seeds, beans, lentils, peas, and fresh raw vegetables.

Natural Prescription for Health: When eating organic produce, leave the washed skin on the apples and eggplant. I would suggest, since eggplant is a nightshade, that you do not eat it more than once or twice a month if you have emotional challenges and anger. The liver is the organ of anger and must be functioning optimally to process the nightshade family.

Personal Thoughts/Goals:

_____

_____

_____

_____

Day 164

A Vegetable Garden

For the land which you go to possess is not like the land of Egypt from which you have come, where you sowed your seed and watered it by foot, as a vegetable garden (Deuteronomy 11:10).

Bible-time people literally died for a vegetable garden. Jezebel had Naboth murdered so her husband, Ahab, could have a vegetable garden in First Kings 21:2. God gave Adam a garden. After He was crucified, Jesus was laid in a garden tomb. Gardens are good for you physically and emotionally. I have patients who spend hours in their gardens. It is very therapeutic. Then at the end of the season, there is much pleasure in giving away the fruits of your love and toil.

Plan ahead and shop early for your plants. Buy seeds and grow seedlings for planting after all signs of frost. Leaf lettuce is easy to grow, and it produces for several months during the late spring and early summer. Choose different types of yellow and green beans that you can freeze in the fall. Be aware of the different varieties of vine and bush plants. Give yourself enough room for growing cucumbers and tomatoes. Cone-shaped screens that limit spread are great for tight spaces. My suggestion: Decide what you want to grow; then find an organic source of plants and seeds. For fertilizer, I have a source for aged manure. There is always someone who has animal fertilizer. Organic mixtures are readily available today as well.

Natural Prescription for Health: Find a sunny location for your garden. Obtain quality soil and add compost throughout the year. Put the residue from juicing in your compost.

Personal Thoughts/Goals:

_____

_____

_____

_____

Day 165

Castor Oil Pack

So he went to him and bandaged his wounds, pouring on oil and wine; and he set him on his own animal, brought him to an inn, and took care of him (Luke 10:34).

Oil can be a healing agent for many conditions. The properties in God-made organic, natural oil are best (no solvents in the refining process). I generally eat flax and olive oil daily. From my experience helping even the most serious health conditions, I have found the oil processing liver to be a pivotal factor for restoring health. We use a low-tech, low-budget protocol fondly called the "castor oil pack." (See pages 224–225.) Castor oil itself has natural healing physiology. It contains natural levels of pain-relieving, health-promoting fat tissue hormones called Prostaglandin 3 (PG3).

Put castor oil on a piece of wool—we use unbleached lamb's wool—and warm it in the oven for ten minutes at three hundred degrees. Place a heating pad in a plastic bag, and cover the floor or couch with plastic or a towel. Dress in a set of clothes that you don't mind getting oily. Put the warm castor-oiled wool on your lower right rib cage and belly. Put the heating pad (high setting) on top of the wool for one hour. Rest. Apply this castor oil pack once a week for six months. You can do it as often as you like after that. This procedure revitalizes liver function. Remember to drink water and avoid toxic food and beverages.

Natural Prescription for Health: Weekly castor oil pack application to the liver area promotes function. (Check with your healthcare provider before using the castor oil pack.)

Personal Thoughts/Goals:

_____

_____

_____

_____

Day 166

Every Part Does Its Share

…Christ—from whom the whole body, joined and knit together by what every joint supplies, according to the effective working by which every part does its share, causes growth of the body for the edifying of itself in love (Ephesians 4:15-16).

High-speed Internet is impressive. How did we ever get along without cell phones, scanners, Twitter, Facebook, and the Cloud? God created the body to be one contiguous unit with a spectacular communication system called the nervous system. One unit—totally working together as the Body of Christ working in harmony. Every part of the body depends on the other systems.

Liver congestion from poor diet choices, including lymph-plugging dairy, results in acne and other skin lesions. Sugar and dairy consumption can create referred pain to the left shoulder blade and neck. Constipation can lead to headaches. Signs of a stressed thyroid are thinning hair and yellow teeth. Yeast overgrowth resulting from too many antibiotics can precipitate fungus around the nails. Gallbladder congestion often precipitates right knee and right shoulder pain. A misaligned vertebra compresses delicate spinal nerves leading to impaired bodily function. Forty-six percent of patients with digestive distress have mid-back strain, irritating the vertebrae involved with stomach function.

Natural Prescription for Health: Regular bowel elimination two hours after a meal is normal. Constipation is a sign of poor function. Drink water, eat fiber.

Personal Thoughts/Goals:

_____

_____

_____

_____

Day 167

Fasting to Focus

But after long abstinence from food, then Paul stood in the midst of them... (Acts 27:21).

Jesus told His disciples that prayer and fasting are necessary in some situations to see a move of God. Do you live to eat or eat to live? Look at America today. What do you see? Most Americans look like they live to eat. In the Bible, Jesus often talks about fasting. And in Matthew 6:16-18, He taught that people should not let others know that they are fasting—with drawn faces.

Fasting promotes digestive tract rest. I have fasted with vegetable broth and a plant-based protein supplement for up to two weeks. An easily digested protein will help prevent muscle breakdown. Generally it may take up to twenty-four hours for your body to adjust without hunger pains. Make sure you drink plenty of water. You may have a caffeine or sugar withdrawal headache; blood vessels will be pounding. You can lose up to fourteen pounds in two weeks. Focusing on God's Word and prayer time will increase your sensitivity to the Holy Spirit.

Natural Prescription for Health: Limit food choices to fruit and vegetables for three days for your first fast.

Personal Thoughts/Goals:

_____

_____

_____

_____

Day 168

Raising Bran

Men who consume more bran have a lower risk of heart disease.

In a study of more than forty-two thousand men, those who typically ate at least seven grams of bran a day had a thirty percent lower risk of coronary heart disease than those who consumed no bran.

While men who consumed more whole grains also had a lower risk, the link with bran was stronger. (Earlier studies showed a lower risk in women who ate more whole grains.)

Although the bran eaters had fiber-rich diets, the researchers suggest that it's not the fiber alone, but the vitamins, minerals, plant estrogens, or antioxidants in bran and whole grains that help protect the heart.[28]

Natural Prescription for Health: Eat more whole grains, especially bran cereals that are high in fiber (at least five grams per serving). They're usually a richer source of fiber than bran muffins, wheat bran bread, oat bran bread, or whole-wheat bread.

> I never complained about being constipated because for as long as I can remember, it's been a part of my life. I regularly purchased over-the-counter laxatives, stool softeners, and Fleets (an at-home enema product). Due to the weekly chiropractic adjustments to my spine, my bowel movements are regular and come with ease. I am no longer dependent on laxatives. I also eat more "live" foods such as fresh vegetables and fruit and drink lots of water (which hasn't been that easy) due to Dr. DeMaria's encouragement. If anyone is tired of battling health challenges, I recommend all-natural, alternative care. —Mary Skinner

Personal Thoughts/Goals:

_____

_____

_____

_____

Oils and Toils

Media-driven medical information has fueled health awareness in America, but the media doesn't routinely inform the public about *nutritional* health. Instead of the medicines touted for health, your body needs oil and fat to operate at peak performance; low-fat, fat-free foods leave your body in a deficient state. Focus on balancing your meals to include items prepared with olive oil, which can be heated to moderate temperatures. Flax oil, a common but deficient oil in our culture, promotes heart and brain health. Flax oil actively reduces pain and should not be heated. Start taking a quality, organic flax oil product today. A logical amount is one tablespoon per one hundred pounds of body weight. Do not heat flax oil.

It is possible to have the Omega 3 and Omega 6 oils and their precursors assessed. Optimal oil function and physiology are necessary for cell function. You may be unknowingly suffering from hormonal challenges, including hot flashes, dry skin, fatigue, and depression because you are using the inappropriate oil for *your* body. We use a simple blood test to assess our patients' levels and commonly notice a lack of Omega 3 oils, low zinc levels, and too much Omega 6 and trans fat. You can go to www.druglessdoctor.com for details on how you can receive a kit sent directly to your home to be forwarded on to a lab.

Castor Oil Pack

Recommendation: With the approval of your physician, you may use the Castor Oil Pack whenever you so desire or feel a need.

Castor Oil Packs have been employed for health benefits for centuries. Reportedly, they were used in ancient India, China, Persia, Egypt, Africa, Greece, Rome, and in North and South America. More modern medical literature indicates their use as a treatment for gastrointestinal problems, lacerations, skin disorders such as psoriasis, as an evacuant, and as a vehicle for introducing medications into the body. Common usage had been for improving elimination capacities, stimulating the liver and gallbladder, healing lesions and adhesions, relief of pain, reduction of inflammation, increasing lymphatic circulation and drawing acids and poisons out of bodily tissues. Generally speaking, you may wish to employ them to assist your body in its healing efforts in any of these areas.

Necessary Items:

- Castor Oil (one hundred percent pure, cold-pressed)

- Wool Flannel (Cotton flannel should not be used)

- Heating Pad

Procedure:

- Fold the wool flannel so that it is three or four layers thick.

- Saturate the wool flannel with castor oil.

- Place the saturated wool flannel in a baking dish and heat slowly in the oven so that the pad becomes hot, but not too hot to place on your skin. (Set your oven on low heat and watch your pad carefully and frequently, so as not to burn it.)

- Rub some oil into the skin on your abdomen.

- Lay the warm—not too hot—wool flannel over your abdomen.

- Cover with saran wrap or plastic.

- Cover with a heating pad for one hour. (It is important to keep the area as hot as possible. This is why a heating pad is recommended instead of a hot water bottle. A hot water bottle cools too quickly and does not maintain a consistent, very hot temperature.)

- When finished, remove the flannel and wash your skin.

- Store the flannel in your baking dish covered with saran wrap or in a zip lock bag. It does not have to be refrigerated. Castor oil is very stable and does not go rancid like other oils do.

- If the flannel becomes discolored, other than the normal color of the oil on it, it is probably due to the drawing of toxins out of the body. When this occurs, wash or discard the flannel.

The flannel can be left on for longer periods if desired. A typical use cycle would be three consecutive days per week for as long as is needed. It can be done more often if desired.

Day 169

Time for an Oil Change

...How long will you mourn for Saul, seeing I have rejected him from reigning over Israel? Fill your horn with oil and go... (1 Samuel 16:1).

Samuel was quite beside himself when Saul was disobedient in his behavior. The Lord told Samuel to get going with new oil in his horn. Vehicles need to have the oil changed on a regular maintenance plan to function at one hundred percent efficiency. Thick, old, dirty, rancid oil creates friction and blown gaskets.

Your body requires oil to function. There are two critical oils your body cannot make on its own, called essential fatty acids. Clinical-based evidence from diet journaling suggests we get more than enough of the Omega 6 essential fats from snack foods. Even supposedly "healthy" expeller pressed oils such as safflower and sunflower can create an imbalance when too much is consumed.

Samuel more than likely used olive oil. Olive oil is great on salads, breads, and for sautéing, and it should be used in a rotation of oil choices. I strongly encourage flax oil—which needs to be refrigerated, never heated, and is an excellent source of Omega 3 fats. Flax oil is not commonly used in most meal planning. One tablespoon daily per one hundred pounds is a good place to start. Put it on salads, breads, potatoes, rice, or straight up.

Natural Prescription for Health: Omega 6-rich safflower, sunflower, primrose, borage, and black currant oils can be transformed into painful arachidonic acid when consumed consistently. Use olive oil and flax oil, in addition to other healthy oils.

Personal Thoughts/Goals:

_____

_____

_____

_____

Day 170

Flax for All Occasions

…But she [Rahab] *had brought them up to the roof and hid them with the stalks of flax, which she had laid…on the roof…* (Joshua 2:6).

Food items show up in the most unusual places—like on the roof. Flax has been used for a variety of purposes over the centuries.

Flax seeds are pressed oil, one of the two essential oils needed for the body to thrive. Flax, also called linseed oil, goes through steps to make two other fats called DHA or EPA. EPA is a fat that is used by the body to help promote heart and blood vessel health. DHA is important to support brain and nervous system health.

I have seen patients with depression, headaches, anxiety, ADHD, and other conditions improve by consuming one tablespoon of flax oil per one hundred pounds of body weight. This is a winner of a supplement!

Natural Prescription for Health: Two teaspoons of Sardine/Anchovy Bio-Omega 3 oil every three days (anchovy and sardines are small fish, which means less toxic fat), while avoiding trans fat and sugar, will reduce inflammation naturally without the toxic side effects of medication.

Personal Thoughts/Goals:

_____

_____

_____

_____

Day 171

Human-made Fat Versus God-made Fat

Bring your father and your households and come to me; I will give you the best
of the land of Egypt, and you will eat the fat of the land (Genesis: 45:18).

God made food and drink that people have tampered with; therefore, read the PLU labels on fruits and vegetables and wisely choose the #9 (organic) versus the #8 (genetically-altered) or all other numbers (which will have a herbicide or pesticide application during the growing season). What is found in nature is organic (without human-made herbicides, pesticides, and synthetic hormones or fertilizers) and has all the complex nutrients to be properly processed in the body. I recently read an interesting title for "White Oil." This product has had essentially all the color and nutrients stripped away.

There are fats that are saturated in the animal and plant kingdoms. Sugarcane and hops are in the kingdom, also. Consistent daily consumption of red meat will cause a problem. I am not naïve, and I don't want you to have your head in the sand. Focus on oils in nature. Olive oil, which can be heated, and flax oil, which should not be heated, are affordable, healthy oils. I have incorporated coconut oil in our practice for patients who want to heat an oil at higher temperature without using human-made trans fats.

Ultimately, my advice is to avoid fried foods and to never use trans fat, hydrogenated, or partially hydrogenated fat. Stay away from any human-made oil, regardless of how safe the research says it is. Always be aware of who paid for the research analysis touting a "safe alternative." Synthetic fat interferes with cell membrane function.

Natural Prescription for Health: Vary the source of olive oil. Do not use it for high heating.

Personal Thoughts/Goals:

_____

_____

_____

_____

Day 172

Peter's Fish

...Go to the sea, cast in a hook, and take the fish that comes up first... (Matthew 17:27).

The unknown number of miracles performed, as well as the ones written in God's Word, reveal the vastness of God's humor and personality. Imagine rubbing saliva in dirt and making mud to relieve blindness. Now there's to "mud in your eye"! On our family trip to Israel, I took a fishing pole for one purpose—to catch a "St. Peter" fish, the one that had the coin inside to pay the taxes of Peter and Jesus. My son did catch one fish, but alas, no money this time. It was an awesome experience all the same.

Peter and John must have consumed fish regularly since that was their livelihood. Fish is an excellent source of DHA fat and protein for brain food. Broiled fish or covered and baked fish on the grill is an excellent method of preparing fish dishes. A dash of lemon and fresh herbs add flavor. Avoid deep-fried fish at all costs and do not eat raw fish. Parasite eggs that are microscopic in size can grow into parasites over forty feet long. Parasites eat first and afterward they release toxic excrements. They leave you the leftovers—at best.

Natural Prescription for Health: Add broiled or baked ocean fish to your diet rotation. Outside grilling is my favorite! (Review Day 111 for additional fish information.)

Personal Thoughts/Goals:

_____

_____

_____

_____

Day 173

Pass the Olive Oil

...You shall tread the olives... (Micah 6:15).

The Mediterranean diet, which includes olives and simple complex foods, promotes heart health. Cholesterol levels are similar between the Mediterranean diet and the typical Western plan; however, there are one-third less hospitalizations for heart disease in the Mediterranean diet. Focus more on fresh fruits, nuts, legumes, and whole foods versus Danish, cookies, fries, and convenience packaged items.

Having no plan is a plan to fail. Start planning Mediterranean-style foods in your meals. Be sure to include fresh vegetables, fruit, and organic chicken or turkey. To save money, buy the poultry on sale and freeze it in amounts your family will eat. Try sautéing a variety of vegetables in olive oil—only a spritz—and add Celtic Sea Salt and herbs. Vegetables in olive oil compliment any meal.

Natural Prescription for Health: Use olive oil, basil, and freshly squeezed lemon wedge as a salad dressing on your mixed greens.

Personal Thoughts/Goals:

_____

_____

_____

_____

Day 174

Butter or Margarine?

The words of his mouth were smoother than butter... (Psalm 55:21).

Is butter better than margarine? This question sustains a marketing battle waged in the media by the dairy boards and oil processors. Margarine is a human-made toxic substance that promotes the disease it was supposed to help. So much for that. Butter is a neutral fat, not good and not bad. It is not necessary and in excess is dangerous. Butter is useful for frying because it tolerates high heat and is easy to digest. You can make butter better by adding high oleic safflower or sunflower oil to it and mixing them together for heating. To spread on breads, add flax oil to butter for a flavorful nutty twist.

We generally do not use a lot of butter, but it is available in our home. We never use margarine. Butter is low in the essential fatty acids and has high levels of other fats that compete with flax. One pound of butter does contain one gram of cholesterol, which may be an issue for some who have high cholesterol affected by diet. Butter does not have all the factors in itself to be properly metabolized, and it does have a small amount of natural trans fat.

Natural Prescription for Health: Always choose God-made versus human-made food items.

Personal Thoughts/Goals:

Day 175

Better Than Statins

What lowers LDL ("bad") cholesterol better than statin drugs? Statins *plus* a healthy diet.

Researchers gave 120 men with high cholesterol either the statin drug, Zocor, or a placebo (sugar pill) and instructed them to eat either their usual diet or a Mediterranean-type diet.

The Mediterranean diet was high in fruits and vegetables and low in saturated and *trans* fats (the meat was lean and the cheese, milk, and yogurt were low-fat). The diet replaced the saturated and *trans* fats with unsaturated fats, especially Omega 3 fats (from fish, canola oil, and canola margarine).

After twelve weeks, the diet had cut LDL by eleven percent, Zocor had cut it by thirty percent, and diet plus Zocor cut LDL cholesterol by forty-one percent. A bonus: the Mediterranean diet wiped out the (unwanted) thirteen-percent rise in insulin levels caused by the Zocor.[29] *In our practice, we lower cholesterol up to forty percent by eliminating sugar and eating beets.*

Natural Prescription for Health: Whether or not you take statin drugs, you should eat plenty of fruits and vegetables and replace saturated and *trans* fats (in meats, dairy, and store-bought or restaurant-baked goods and fried foods) with unsaturated fats (in foods such as fish, oils, nuts, salad dressing, and avocado).

> When I first came to see Dr. DeMaria, I had bad hip, leg, and shoulder pain. I had a terrible time sleeping because the pain was so bad! I even took Celebrex for the pain, which did nothing for me. Following the information and care provided by Dr. Bob, I can certainly do a lot more things and for a longer period of time. I now have no pain at night. I am very grateful for his care.
> —Roxine Jones

Personal Thoughts/Goals:

_____

_____

_____

_____

Day 176

Fat Craving Snack Food?

*So he called the name of that place Kibroth Hattaavah, because there they
buried the people who had yielded to craving* (Numbers 11:34).

I believe that people crave food unknowingly. The public is attracted to the preservatives, taste enhancers, and nitrates. The body literally has an endorphin reaction high from the excitotoxin stimulation. Trans fats, partially and totally hydrogenated, are in salty, addictive snack foods. Americans consume approximately twenty-five to thirty pounds of snacks per year.

Trans fat is vegetable oil that has been heated and had hydrogen added. This fat was developed in volume to lower cholesterol levels, but in actuality it raises the LDL cholesterol and lowers the HDL cholesterol. You cannot fool Mother Nature. Trans fat is incorporated into cell membranes causing the cells to become hardened. The metabolism of other fat pathways are sabotaged with trans fat snack food consumption for up to 102 days. ADHD, depression, Alzheimer's, and pain can all result because of trans fat. But don't overdo safflower or sunflower oil for snacks either. Even though they are not trans fat and are healthier, over-consuming these oils can result in pain.

Natural Prescription for Health: Read labels and avoid items containing trans fat. A "low fat" label may actually be a red flag for trans fat or other toxic human-made fat substitutes.

Personal Thoughts/Goals:

_____

_____

_____

_____

Day 177

The Whole World in His Hand

*But now, O Lord, You are our Father; we are the clay, and You are our potter;
and all we are the work of Your hand* (Isaiah 64:8).

God has us in His hand. We are blessed that we have a Heavenly Father who wants a relationship with us. When was the last time you sat quietly, worshiped, and praised God, regardless of your current state? Raise your hands in worship.

Hand and finger pain can be disabling. A common condition I frequently assist is "trigger finger." The tendons located on the palm aspect of your hand can become irritated with small stress centers. This is normally a result of poor fat metabolism due to a whole food B6 deficiency. The body will send what feels like a bean substance as a healing mechanism. This growth can actually get trapped, preventing your finger from relaxing. The result is a snap noise, and it is painful.

Trigger fingers are a symptom of a deeper problem, which is poor metabolism of a fat-like substance for pain relief called prostaglandin 3. You can actually get tendonitis in other areas beside the finger, elbow, wrist, shoulder, hip, ankle, or toe. Consume one tablespoon of flax daily per one hundred pounds and add a whole food B6 to your supplement protocol, 150 milligrams daily.

Natural Prescription for Health: Eliminate trans or partially hydrogenated fat from your diet. They stop the good prostaglandin, PG-3, production.

Personal Thoughts/Goals:

_____

_____

_____

_____

Day 178

Infuse Your Olive Oil

For the Lord your God is bringing you into a good land,...a land of wheat and barley, of vines and fig trees and pomegranates, a land of olive oil and honey (Deuteronomy 8:7-8).

Herbs are discussed from the very beginning of creation. We use herbs in our home year round. My suggestion is go to your health food store and purchase single containers of herbs, one per week. Add them to your salads. Add your favorite herb to the food you prepare near the end of cooking. Adding herbs too soon may deplete the essence due to the warming process. I enjoy basil, dill, parsley, thyme, oregano, and chives.

Periodically I purchase a gallon of olive oil and add a variety of my favorite herbs and sun dried tomatoes to the container. The herbs are absorbed by the oil for three weeks. I pour off the oil into dark, rubber-sealed bottles using a fine sieve or strainer and store the bottles in a dark, cool cupboard or pantry. You will passionately fall in love with the enriched flavor. Olive oil is an excellent source of fat that is good for you. Sauté your favorite vegetables with olive oil over moderate heat. My motto: If Jesus used it, which I am sure He did, so can I.

Natural Prescription for Health: Grow your own herbs—they can be dried for year-round use.

Personal Thoughts/Goals:

_____

_____

_____

_____

Day 179

Depression Is Serious

Truly the light is sweet, and it is pleasant for the eyes to behold the sun
(Ecclesiastes 11:7).

Do not stop any medication without consulting a trained healthcare provider who has experience with antidepressants and natural alternatives. It is not uncommon to read headlines such as, "Sermon Reportedly Upset Shooter." Several church members were killed by a person who had a history of depression. The article reported that the event occurred in the northern US in the winter.

It is my experience that depression is common among individuals who live in dreary, lack-of-sunshine climates. The ability to be outside in the sun impacts your emotional health. Sun helps the emotions by facilitating the movement of fat and minerals, all needed for brain health. I am not promoting sun worshiping or overexposure. I am going to suggest, however, that those who live in cloud-covered areas increase their flax oil during winter months, especially if they have dry, flaky skin. I also recommend a regular exercise program with free-weight resistance training, machines or elastic bands, and aerobic activity. Motion is life and increases the "feel good" endorphins.

Natural Prescription for Health: Add liquid sunshine, flax oil, to your diet, one tablespoon per one hundred pounds of body weight.

Personal Thoughts/Goals:

_____

_____

_____

_____

Day 180

Be a Nut

Moreover the word of the Lord came to me, saying, "Jeremiah, What do you see?" And I said, "I see a branch of an almond tree," Then the Lord said to me, "You have seen well, for I am ready to perform my word" (Jeremiah 1:11-12).

Nuts are an excellent source of protein and good fat. There has been confusion about nuts because of low-fat restricted diets, but I recommend nuts to my patients. Over time even patients with bowel challenges can start eating nuts again.

I generally prepare a small container of raw nuts daily to eat midmorning or afternoon. Protein is to the body what a log is to fire—a slow-burning source of fuel. Raw nuts provide a steady blood sugar response and reduce hunger. Add nuts to your breakfast routine, quinoa, grits, non-gluten, or gluten cereals. I generally eat raw cashews, almonds, and walnuts. Walnuts are not a common "health food topic, but they are a super source of Omega 3 fat. Almonds are a neutral nut, not acidic or alkaline and they add calcium to the system. I also enjoy sesame seeds, which are an excellent source of calcium, and sunflower seeds. Sprinkle the seeds on any item you like. Pumpkin seeds are a good source of zinc. Peanuts are not nuts; they are legumes and can create problems for some.

Natural Prescription for Health: Beware that red or white pistachios are generally overcooked and can be rancid.

Personal Thoughts/Goals:

_____

_____

_____

_____

Day 181

Stop Pain

Before them people writhe in pain; all faces are drained of color (Joel 2:6).

Relentless pain can stop the best of anyone in their tracks. Billions of dollars are spent annually on pain relievers. I am baffled that with all the information on pain relief, you rarely see an article on what *causes* the pain. COX inhibitors, a media term for medication developed to prevent digestive distress while relieving pain, commonly result in death. Billions of dollars are made on millions of prescriptions without hesitation.

Do you want to know what causes most of your pain? *You* do! Yep! You read that right. What you eat either promotes or suppresses fat tissue-like hormones in your body called prostaglandins (PG). PG1 & 3 relieve pain internally by taking it away. PG2 creates pain. The key is how do you raise 1 & 3 and lower 2. In theory, it is not hard. Flax oil, walnuts, greens, and deepwater ocean fish become PG3. Safflower, sunflower, primrose, and black currant become PG1. However, too much consumption of these overflow to number 2. PG2 is from red meat, dairy, and shellfish. Sugar, aspirin, trans fat, and insulin stop or hinder PG1 and 3 and promote PG2. COX 1 and 2 inhibitors, common "modern" pain relievers, hinder PG2—but not without side effects, such as stroke and heart disease. (See *Dr. Bob's Trans Fat Survival Guide* at www.DruglessCare.com)

Natural Prescription for Health: To prevent pain, eliminate sugar, dairy, red meat, and PG1 oil-based snack foods for one month. Add flax (one tablespoon per one hundred pounds daily), with alfalfa tablets (four to six daily).

Personal Thoughts/Goals:

_____

_____

_____

_____

Day 182

Eat Less, Live Longer

Six months of calorie restriction, with or without exercise, lowered two signs of aging in overweight men and women. Researchers assigned forty-eight healthy, sedentary, overweight, (but not obese) people, aged twenty-six to forty-nine, either:

- Twenty-five percent fewer calories than they need

- Twelve and a half percent fewer calories plus enough exercise to burn twelve and a half percent more calories than usual (typically forty-five to fifty minutes of walking, running, or cycling five times a week).

- A very low-calorie diet (890 calories a day) until they lost fifteen percent of their body weight, followed by enough calories to keep their weight constant or their usual diet.

After six months, all but the usual-diet group had lower levels of fasing insulin and core body temperature, which are linked to longer life spans in animals. Furthermore, all but the usual-diet group had less DNA damage, and their bodies adapted to the lower-calorie diets by burning fewer calories. What to do: If you are overweight, there is no question that cutting back calories makes sense.[30]

Natural Prescription for Health: Eat more fruits, vegetables, beans, whole grains, and seafood. Replace saturated fats from meat and dairy with unsaturated fats from oils and nuts.

> Before making Dr. DeMaria's recommended lifestyle changes, my skin would not heal, I had knee pain when I walked or ran, and I had numbness in both hands. I also had visual disturbances and headaches that occurred often. I had also invested in many topicals from dermatologists that didn't help, and I also took oral antibiotics. It has been difficult, but I have eliminated most sugar from my diet and now take a zinc supplement, flax oil, and vitamins. The information provided by Dr. Bob has improved my life. My health has improved and has given me hope for further improvements. I have given my testimony to many friends and family and hope that they find their way here! —Laura Lackas

Personal Thoughts/Goals:

_____

_____

Day 183

Oil Sustains Life

Then the dove came to him [Noah] *in the evening, and behold, a freshly plucked olive leaf was in her mouth...* (Genesis 8:11).

Machines require oil from a quality source to function for long life. We do not have a red light blinking on our foreheads saying, "Check Engine Oil." Our machine uses oil to make hormones, cell membranes, energy, and it even gives taste to food. Dry skin, especially in the winter, is a blinking red light that you need oil.

Fat and oil consumption can be confusing. An excellent oil source for salad dressings and sautéing is olive oil. Olive oil, from an organic source, first pressed without heat or chemical extraction, is an excellent choice.

I do not recommend a low-fat diet. Fat is needed for function in all organs, but don't overdo it. Flax oil on salad is an excellent healthy habit.

Natural Prescription for Health: Try using organic coconut oil on bread or toast, it is an excellent alternative for butter.

Personal Thoughts/Goals:

_____

_____

_____

_____

Day 184

Fat Phobia

So he brought the tribute to Eglon King of Moab. (Now Elgon was a very fat man)
(Judges 3:17).

I am not sure what frightens the public more—eating fat, which causes obesity, or wearing fat, which increases heart attack risk. Fat is necessary for optimal function. Your body sends messages on a layer of fat. Cell membranes are made of fat, and your brain is primarily fat. Fat gives taste to food and has nine calories per gram. In America over the last thirty years, we have avoided fat like the plague, yet people are fatter now than ever. Heart disease and cancer lead the statistics for death, and both of these common conditions are affected by obesity.

So what is up? Low carbohydrate, low fat has meant "low cholesterol" to most, but cholesterol is not even a fat. Your body needs cholesterol in order to function one hundred percent. Your body will make whatever cholesterol is needed. The general population is also low in Omega 3 fats. My suggestion would be to focus on consuming plant-based oils, especially olive and flax oil. Eating red meat periodically, such as one time a week, is acceptable. Avoid sweet fruit and sugar overload—they convert to fat in your body.

Natural Prescription for Health: If low fat includes "human-made" on the label—avoid it.

Personal Thoughts/Goals:

_____

_____

_____

_____

Day 185

Can Oil Be Soft?

...His words were softer than oil... (Psalm 55:21).

The human body needs oil to operate efficiently, much like any other piece of machinery. Cell membranes in the body are made up of different types of fats, oil, and cholesterol. Saturated fat is firm, or hard, at room temperature and creates hardness in the walls of blood vessels. The term saturation comes from the way fat atoms and molecules are connected. Fats that are unsaturated with several connections or links holding the atoms and molecules together are softer and more pliable.

Heating oils alters the makeup and causes damage. I encourage my patients to avoid foods fried in high temperature oils. America's lower state of health is partly caused by consuming heated oils.

You can improve the softness of blood vessel walls by using flax or olive oil.

Natural Prescription for Health: Consume one tablespoon of organic flax oil daily. This is equivalent to approximately twelve capsules.

Personal Thoughts/Goals:

_____

_____

_____

_____

Day 186

Dandruff—Head Skin Itch

If a man or woman has a sore [or skin itch] *on the head…* (Leviticus 13:29).

Inflammation of the scalp and head can be quite annoying. Billions of dollars are spent each year on shampoos designed to *control* exfoliation of skin on top of the head. Watch for chemicals that you are applying to your brain, which is adjacent to the skull. The scalp and tissues around the head and face are rich with blood vessels. Sodium lauryl sulfate, a common toxic ingredient, is going to be absorbed, evenly slightly, and over time there will be an accumulation, causing liver congestion.

I treat most patients with dandruff, seborrhea, and eczema with a balance of oils. The oils should have a combination of the Omega 6 and Omega 3 fats. Generally patients are deficient in the Omega 3 fats such as flax oil. For whatever reason, dandruff responds more effectively to a product we use called BioOmega with a combination of Omega 3 oils. Skin inflammation, just as other body inflammations, responds with the right oil. Read product ingredient labels on all lotions you apply to your skin. Avoid sodium lauryl sulfate.

Natural Prescription for Health: One tablespoon of a balance of Omega 6 & 3 oils per one hundred pounds of body weight will heal dry skin challenges.

Personal Thoughts/Goals:

_____

_____

_____

_____

Day 187

Avoid Pain

Yet, I am glad now, not because you were pained, but because you were pained into repentance, [and so turned you to God]... (2 Corinthians 7:9 AMP).

Emotional pain can be a motivator for repentance. Paul, writing to the church in Corinth, knew that their pain was instrumental in motivating them to change direction. It has been estimated that eighty-six million Americans have some type of physical pain.[31] Pain is a sign of inflammation. People avoid pain by taking pain relieving meds that do not get to the cause of pain. Do you know you can minimize or eliminate pain on your own without the bad or near-death side effects from pain relieving medications?

First, the leading cause of pain is the improper metabolism of a tissue fat hormone called prostaglandin 3, or PG3. PG3 production is interrupted by lack of vitamins and minerals, especially B vitamins, zinc, and magnesium. Second, the leading factor depleting these important ingredients is stress and sugar. What should you do? Delete sugar from your diet, reduce stress (exercise helps), and take PG3-promoting flax oil— one tablespoon per one hundred pounds of body weight.

Natural Prescription for Health: Got pain? Get flax! Add it to your salads and veggies. Do not heat flax; add it to already prepared entrees.

Personal Thoughts/Goals:

_____

_____

_____

_____

Day 188

Butter Is Better

So he took butter and milk and the calf which he had prepared, and set it before them; and he stood by them under the tree as they ate (Genesis 18:8).

Butter is God-made. Margarine is human-made. Is butter better than margarine? As mentioned previously, this question sustains a marketing battle waged in the media by dairy boards and oil processors. There are about five hundred different fatty acids that have been isolated from butter, which are easy to digest. A pound of butter contains one gram of cholesterol, which is required by all of our cells. Butter does have trans fat, and it is more easily metabolized than trans fat found in hydrogenated oils. Butter can be used for frying and other high heat applications because it is mainly saturated. Butter is a neutral fat, not good or bad. Use organic-sourced butter without pesticides and antibiotics.

Margarine is created by heating vegetable oil to high temperatures and adding hydrogen to it. The oil becomes trans fatty acid and interferes with cell membrane configuration. Margarine interferes with good essential fat in the body, which causes pain. It raises LDL cholesterol, which is a sign that it creates inflammation.

Now ask yourself, which is better!

Natural Prescription for Health: Blend a tablespoon of olive, safflower, or sunflower oil with room temperature organic butter for a better butter.

Personal Thoughts/Goals:

_____

_____

_____

_____

Day 189

Healthy Diets, Healthy Hearts

Heart disease rates in women have dropped, and changes in diet, smoking cigarettes, and the use of estrogen explain much of the decline, say researchers at the Harvard School of Public Health.

Frank Hu and colleagues compared the health and lifestyles of roughly eighty-six thousand women in the Nurses' Health Study. Between 1980 and 1994, the incidence of heart disease dropped thirty-one percent. Diet explained roughly half (sixteen percent) of the decline, while a drop in smoking accounted for thirteen percent, and the increased use of estrogen by postmenopausal women explained nine percent.

Among the dietary changes, the women ate less *trans* and saturated fat, more polyunsaturated vegetable and fish oils, more fiber from breads, grains, and cereals, and more folate (a B-vitamin).

But a rise in obesity offset some of the gains. "If obesity hadn't increased, the decline in heart disease would have been much greater," says Hu.[32]

> When I first came to see Dr. DeMaria, I had very bad sinus problems. I was also taking blood pressure medication. The information provided by Dr. Bob has made me more aware of the value of what goes into my mouth and how it affects my entire body. I have greatly reduced my sugar intake, and I also use flax oil daily along with fresh carrot juice. Yum! Staying away from processed food has been difficult. It is so easy to grab and eat; however, I do not get any nutritional value from it. As a result from making a few lifestyle changes, I hardly notice any problems at all! There are so many people who are my age with so many aches and pains due to their diet and I almost have none! I feel really good about my maintenance care from Dr. Bob. —Rebecca Szilagyi

Personal Thoughts/Goals:

_____

_____

_____

_____

Optimal Health for Women

Females live on a fine line of hormonal balance. Any overload or deficiency can create a cascade of symptoms. A leading cause of female issues is estrogen overload. The liver is the clearing house for hormone function. Childbearing creates additional stress on the operating function. Women who focus on whole food diets, exercise, and detoxification live healthier lives.

Men, read this section to increase your wisdom about female health. The natural principles affect you too. You may consider reading the bestselling *Dr. Bob's Drugless Guide to Balancing Female Hormones*.

Many people spend more time preparing for a party or special event than they do their future. I suggest that over the next sequence you use the blank pages provided at the back of the book and write down your one-month, six-month, and twelve-month goals. Also, plan five- and ten-year projection goals. I suggest you focus on some of the patterns discussed up to this point, plus skill set enhancement, financial, personal, and relationship goals.

Day 190

Balancing Human Hormones

If a woman has a discharge of blood for many days, other than a part of her customary...
(Leviticus 15:25).

The woman with the issue of blood had a hormone imbalance that precipitated heavy flow. Proper liver function is critical in keeping estrogen balanced with progesterone. Elevated estrogen is challenging to deal with today due to the addition of human-made, synthetic compounds called xenohormones, which mimic estrogen. Our toxic environment with excess xenohormones increases estrogen in a female, disabling the liver from clearing the estrogen. B vitamins are necessary for this process. Sugar and stress deplete B vitamins while snack foods, processed convenience meals, partially hydrogenated or trans fats, and prescription medication can stress an already overworked liver.

The ovaries normally produce enough progesterone when they are functioning but may not be able to keep up the pace when xenohormones are not cleared from the liver fast enough. We supplement with an herb called Chaste Tree for a short time to assist ovary function. I also encourage our female and male patients to incorporate organic iodine to their daily regime. I currently take twelve milligrams daily; start with three to six milligrams daily and slowly progress to twelve milligrams. Increasing progesterone, clearing estrogen, and decreasing sugar helps prevent menstrual headaches and symptoms of PMS. It has also been my observation that miscarriages are associated with low progesterone levels.

Natural Prescription for Health: Eat beets to support liver function.

Personal Thoughts/Goals:

_____

_____

_____

_____

Day 191

Feeling Stressed?

You will keep in perfect peace all who trust in you, all whose thoughts are fixed on you!
(Isaiah 26:3 NLT).

It may surprise you to learn that not all stress is bad. In fact, some stress is very beneficial. What determines whether it is good or bad is how much stress you are under. A little stress can be good. Think of it as tuning a stringed instrument—too tight and it breaks; too little and it is dull.

There are stages of being stressed. The alarm stage is when the original stress occurs. For instance, someone yells "fire" and you run. Today we have people yelling "fire" at us constantly. Over time, the body wears down, and you slip into the resistance stage. Frequent alarms precipitate chronic illness and marital, adult, parent, and child issues. You may develop feelings of hopelessness and helplessness. These feelings lead to exhaustion, along with painful joints, allergies, and more bacterial and viral infections. The physical body is always sick and generally has no sexual desire. You can experience weight gain and low blood sugar with exhaustive stress.

Focus on modifying the stress factors. Add adrenal tissue support, whole foods, pantothenic acid, and vitamin C to your life. Do not overcommit to responsibilities.

Natural Prescription for Health: Limit your commitments outside the home and exercise.

Personal Thoughts/Goals:

_____

_____

_____

_____

Day 192

Detoxified for Health

...Blessed...[are] *the breasts which nursed You!* (Luke 11:27).

Healthy breast tissue is a sign of clear digestive and detoxification function. Just mentioning the word breast cyst or blocked milk duct can send chills down the spine. Thirty percent of American women have fibrocystic breast disease, a benign (noncancerous) condition characterized by round lumps that move freely within the breast tissue. These lumps are usually tender to the touch. In contrast, a cancerous growth in the breast is often not tender or freely movable when touched. The texture of the lumps can vary from soft to firm. For many women, the tenderness may increase as menstruation approaches. Often the cysts fill with fluid and can enlarge premenstrually in response to the increase in hormonal levels during this time.[33]

There are many thoughts and hypothesis by Western medical thinkers as to the cause of breast lesions. Studying natural therapeutics for over thirty years, I must tell you from my experience that the three leading causes of unchecked elevated estrogen levels arise from 1) synthetic HRT (sourced from horse urine), 2) congested livers not capable of clearing estrogen, and 3) obesity. Eating high-fiber food and whole food B vitamins are absolutely necessary to combat high estrogen levels. An optimally functioning thyroid is needed to have proper bowel movements. Flax oil, rich in Omega 3 fat, promotes overall optimal hormonal function. A congested liver from consuming too much caffeine from coffee, tea, and chocolate can also lead to breast cysts.

Keep your liver clean. Eat beets daily. Increase fiber to help assist removal of elevated estrogen. *Do not panic!* Just make some changes.

Natural Prescription for Health: Eat fiber with each meal. Your bowels will move better tomorrow.

Iodine supplementation is critically important today for optimal function for all the cells in the body. Iodine is necessary not only for thyroid utilization; it is also used and needed by the ovaries, breasts, and testes in men. There is a group of elements in the iodine or halide family called bromine, fluorine, and chlorine. These three compete with iodine, often disrupting the position of iodine at the cellular level. We live in a very toxic environment, with an abundance of chlorine when we shower and swim, fluorine when we drink water or brush our teeth, and bromine in white bread and sports drinks.

When the thyroid gland or gas pedal does not have enough iodine, subpar function can occur, and you will have symptoms that include cold hands and feet, constipation, fatigue, yellow teeth, thin sparse hair, depression, and elevated cholesterol levels. The most scientific way to assess your thyroid gland is to have your healthcare provider request the following tests; TSH, T3, and T4 plus a TPO. I also suggest a urine iodine loading test. Optimal thyroid function is one of the many steps you can do to prevent long term chronic health problems.

Personal Thoughts/Goals:

_____

_____

_____

_____

Day 193

What Is in Your Candle?

*As smoke is driven away, so drive them away; as **wax** melts before the fire...*
(Psalm 68:2, emphasis added).

The bee is one of the most uniquely designed creatures on earth. The size of the body in comparison to the wing span would logically suggest that flying is out of the question. God in His infinite wisdom gave us the bee to continue the existence of plants that require pollination. Without bees, our landscape would have a lot less color. Bees work diligently for a season and actually inflict intense fear in individuals who are allergic to their sting. The hard work they do is a benefit to us.

Honey is one of God's ways to bless us with natural sweetness. The wax in the honeycomb provides one of the safest sources of material to make candles. Read the ingredients on candle labels to determine the chemicals, fragrances, and composition of candles commonly featured in novelty and retail outlets. Do the candles you have burn a black smoke? Do your candles have a synthetic fragrance? I know from experience that my air purifier can be rendered useless in a short time when burning petrochemical-based candles.

Natural Prescription for Health: Burn candles made with beeswax.

Personal Thoughts/Goals:

_____

_____

_____

_____

Day 194

Absorbable Calcium

But where can wisdom be found? And where is the place of understanding?...
*No mention shall be made of **coral** or quartz. For the price of wisdom is above rubies*
(Job 28:12,18, emphasis added).

Calcium is a foundation mineral in the framework of our bone structure. The skeletal system is the attachment for tendons, ligaments, and muscles. Organs suspended in the body cavity depend on a secure, firm bone matrix. In my experience, the vertebrae can be indented by cartilage disc material. Patients who smoke appear to have weak bone structure. I am of the opinion that aspirin is not a safe medication. It disrupts body physiology and will slow fracture repair.

Calcium is needed by the bony framework like limestone in concrete. Focus on calcium that is easily absorbed. *Calcium lactate or citrate are assimilated by the digestive system easier than calcium carbonate from oyster shells or coral.* I encourage my female patients to take flax oil and to participate in resistance exercises, as well as avoid sugar and soda.

Remember, sunshine helps calcium absorption. God put the sun in the sky to give life. However, don't overdo it.

Natural Prescription for Health: Plant food is a quality source of useable calcium. Sesame seeds, almonds, and mixed greens are on top of the list.

Personal Thoughts/Goals:

_____

_____

_____

_____

Day 195

Beauty Is Only Skin Deep

...And from the roof he [David] *saw a woman bathing, and the woman was very beautiful to behold* (2 Samuel 11:2).

Beauty is only skin deep. The appearance of skin reveals much about the body physically. In First Samuel 17:42, David, a youth ready to fight Goliath, was *"ruddy and good looking."* Later in his life, he was curious about the appearance of Bathsheba— her beauty caught his attention.

An alarming number of my female patients have what is described as "spider veins" or "spider nevi," which are often found with patients experiencing varicose veins. Cosmetically, they appear as larger areas of engorged blood vessels located usually on the thigh or calf. My clinical experience suggests several possible causative factors. One is that the liver is congested from poor diet choices—sugar, trans fat, and dairy. Varicose veins, common in men and women with congested livers, can create cosmetic and physical issues. Pregnancy, also a stress on the female liver, can cause varicose or spider veins.

Another reason for varicose veins is a deficiency of whole food B vitamins. Your body needs B vitamins to process estrogen. Perimenopausal women generally have high estrogen levels. We use an herb in our practice called Collinsonia Root, along with liver cleansing, to relieve the distress caused by varicose veins.

Natural Prescription for Health: Add a wedge of lemon to morning hot water; then eat the lemon. Eat beets daily and take your whole food B vitamins.

Personal Thoughts/Goals:

_____

_____

_____

_____

Day 196

Nuts to Diabetes

Women who ate nuts at least five times a week had a thirty percent lower risk of diabetes than women who almost never ate nuts reported in a study of more than eighty-three thousand nurses. (Eating nuts one to four times a week or eating peanut butter at least five times a week was linked to a twenty percent lower risk.)[34]

It's not clear whether nuts lower the risk of diabetes because they're high in magnesium, unsaturated fats, or fiber or whether something else about nut-eaters lowers their risk. The researchers took into account the fact that the nut-eaters ate healthier diets, were less likely to smoke and be overweight, and were more likely to exercise. But they may have missed something else about nut-eaters that made them healthier.

Natural Prescription for Health: It's worth adding small servings of nuts to your diet; just keep in mind that they are calorie-dense, so you can't eat them without removing something else. (The study's authors recommend deleting some refined grains and red meat.) There is 150-185 calories in a one-ounce serving of dry roasted nuts. That's just twenty-two almonds or fourteen walnut halves.

> I first came to see Dr. DeMaria because I had back pain. I also had been experiencing an irregular menstrual cycle (spotting and heavy flow). Following Dr. Bob's recommendations, I have eliminated dairy products and now include some supplements in my diet. It has been difficult managing my schedule to include weekly visits to Dr. Bob; however, I would say that Dr. DeMaria has been one of the most influential people in my life in the last ten years. —Georgia Sweeney

Personal Thoughts/Goals:

_____

_____

_____

_____

Day 197

Blessed Is the Womb

...Blessed is the womb that bore You... (Luke 11:27).

The value of a healthy womb is priceless. Jesus spent nine months in Mary's womb prior to entering the world. Multiple children were born to Mary after Him, and they were blessed just because they spent nine months growing where Jesus developed. Wow, that is something to meditate on.

I see a variety of conditions in my practice. Fibroids and heavy menstrual flow are very common in our toxic society. Why does a toxic environment impact the uterus? Because estrogen clearing is delayed in the liver. Your liver processes estrogen with the help of quality B vitamins. There is an excessive amount of xenohormones present in human-made fabric, chemicals, wall coverings, and pollution. Xenohormones mimic estrogen. Estrogen needs to be balanced by progesterone. Stress on the adrenal glands and ovaries diminishes progesterone production. Estrogen, when not balanced by progesterone, activates receptors, which can result in a fibroid and heavy bleeding.

Avoiding sugar, trans fat, alcohol, and even some prescription medications will go a long way to improving uterus health and entire body health.

Natural Prescription for Health: Increase whole food B vitamins found in grains. Eat beets, eliminate trans fats, and add Calcium D Glucarate, known to assist optimal liver function.

Personal Thoughts/Goals:

_____

_____

_____

_____

Day 198

Extreme Menstrual Flow

If a woman has a discharge of blood many days, **other** *than at the time of her customary impurity, or if it runs beyond her usual time…* (Leviticus 15:25, emphasis added).

The leading cause of heavy or extensive menstrual flow is poor diet choices and stress. Stress depletes the body of badly needed whole food B vitamins that are necessary to process estrogen. The liver is programmed to create chemicals to handle the additional emotional load. Fast-paced lifestyles along with emotional highs and lows create additional overload on a liver that is already at its maximum output. Realize also that stress interrupts intestinal absorption. B vitamins are produced in the intestine. Colon irritation also impairs production.

Ladies, before deciding to have a hysterectomy, my suggestion is to first focus on a detoxification program and lifestyle pattern change. Take the words *Danish, cookie, soda, glass of wine,* and so forth out of your vocabulary. Avoid items that are processed. They create additional work on your filter system. You need to increase your consumption of whole food B vitamins, drink more water, take flax, and eat beets.

Natural Prescription for Health: Milk products congest lymphatic flow. Drink water and exercise aerobically.

Personal Thoughts/Goals:

_____

_____

_____

_____

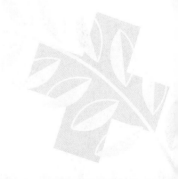

Day 199

Optimal Bone Health

O dry bones, hear the word of the Lord! (Ezekiel 37:4).

Every structure needs a foundation to support it. The human frame and skeleton are made of bone, cartilage, muscles, ligaments, and tendons.

Osteoporosis, or loss of calcium from bone, creates a state of fragility. I encourage my patients to eat consistent, adequate amounts of protein with which bone is inter-mixed in the matrix. A quality source of Omega 3 oil or flax oil is also important to maintain proper hormone function, especially of the thyroid to ensure calcium integrity.

When was the last time you saw an adult cow eating cottage cheese, milk, or ice cream? Cows eat hay, grass, and alfalfa for their sources of calcium. Excellent sources of calcium for you include sesame seeds, mixed greens, almonds, and alfalfa. Keep in mind that eating sugar depletes body calcium.

Natural Prescription for Health: Eat plant or limited animal protein several times daily as a foundation for bone matrix. Thyroid medication when used over time by menopausal women to treat their subpar thyroid function may result in osteoporosis.

Personal Thoughts/Goals:

_____

_____

_____

_____

Day 200

Seasonal Emotions

For the day of the Lord…is at hand: a day of darkness and gloominess,
a day of clouds and thick darkness… (Joel 2:1-2 NKJV).

Darkness is generally associated with negative emotions. *"In Him was life, and the life was the light of men. And the light shines in the darkness, and the darkness did not comprehend it"* (John 1:4-5). Some people become more depressed in the winter months when the days are shorter and darker. I also see an emotional change in some patients around the third week of August. It may be sadness from children leaving for school, a change in the sun pattern, or anticipation of the winter cabin fever. This emotional state is real.

I encourage my clientele who live in the North to exercise daily and to enjoy the sunshine whenever possible. The pineal gland in your brain is affected by sunlight. I discourage sunglasses. They block precious sunlight to your retina. Increase potassium for adrenal support so your eyes will be less bothered by light. Cucumbers and alfalfa are excellent sources of potassium. We recommend a supplement called phosphatidyl choline. This supplement helps break down fats and is beneficial for people with memory loss, depression, and seasonal affect disorder (SAD). I usually see excellent results when patients take six to nine tablets daily.

Natural Prescription for Health: Flax oil, protein, and vitamin B6 assist the body in producing brain-bathing acetylcholine. Include these critical factors in your diet plan.

Personal Thoughts/Goals:

_____

_____

_____

_____

Day 201

Vitamin D Is Free

The sun also rises, and the sun goes down, and hastens to the place where it arose
(Ecclesiastes 1:5).

When the Lord gives you life-sustaining gifts—like oxygen, water, and sun—they are provided freely and abundantly. In ignorance, people are creating an ecosystem that is limiting the supply of all three. We buy water, have limited oxygen in some areas, and have been advised to limit sun exposure.

The Lord put the sun in the sky for a purpose. One of the roles of the sun is to convert the cholesterol in your skin to vitamin D. Vitamin D is critical for optimal calcium absorption. Announcements in magazines, journals, and newspapers suggest we are in a vitamin D deficiency pattern in the US. My advice to patients is to enjoy the morning and evening sun. Think of sun as a natural cholesterol-lowering medication and an osteoporosis supplement. The sun is your friend. Consuming trans fat or hydrogenated fat interferes with the skin/calcium/cholesterol interaction. Take extra flax and calcium when you increase sun exposure.

Natural Prescription for Health: Read labels on suntan lotion. Avoid products containing sodium lauryl sulfate ingredients.

Personal Thoughts/Goals:

_____

_____

_____

_____

Day 202

"I Shall Be Made Well"

Immediately the fountain of her blood was dried up... (Mark 5:29).

The woman with the twelve-year issue of blood, with physician treatment, is becoming a common scenario in our time as well. Evidence-based research suggests that high estrogen levels are the precipitating cause. Saliva hormone evaluation is an excellent screen to evaluate female hormones.

I encourage my patients to eat whole food B vitamins. They are essential to help the liver process estrogen properly. Meal tip: Organic beets, grated raw, on a mixed green salad with quality flax oil; or diced beets baked at 400 degrees, slightly covered with olive oil, promotes liver function.

Avoid items that congest the body's detoxifying organ such as sugar, human-made fats, alcohol, and excessive dairy. Processed food, prescription medications, and stress can also interfere with the liver's activity.

Natural Prescription for Health: Human-made food, beverages, and medications create liver stress. Focus on God-made.

Personal Thoughts/Goals:

_____

_____

_____

_____

Day 203

Eat Your Vegetables

Women who consumed more vegetables (including cauliflower, broccoli, cabbage, onions, squash, and tomatoes) or salad had a lower risk of non-Hodgkin's lymphoma in a study of thirteen hundred people. Fiber was also linked to a lower risk, while eating more fruit (apples and oranges) wasn't.[35]

Natural Prescription for Health: This study doesn't prove that vegetables protect the lymph system. But eating more can't hurt and may reduce your risk of stroke and heart disease, as well as some cancers other than lymphoma.

> My past health complaints ranged from neck and shoulder pain, low back pain, unpleasant periods (cramps, headaches), and just a general feeling of unhealthiness and stress. I wasn't taking any medications; however, with a family history of cancer, heart disease, diabetes, and high blood pressure, having a healthy future looked grim for me.
>
> The care and information provided by Dr. DeMaria has radically changed my life for the *better*. The information provided by Dr. DeMaria is *invaluable* and is the recipe for optimal health. Following his advice, I watch what I eat (especially reducing sugar, dairy, and wheat), and I try to include organic foods and whole food supplements. It has been difficult reducing my intake of sugar and adding exercise to my health regimen, but the most difficult was changing my mindset and lifestyle.
>
> Information is a wonderful thing—but if you do not use the knowledge and put it into practice, it is worthless. Dr. DeMaria provides the knowledge, yet he also provides the continued encouragement to help his patients live optimally! —Brenda Traxtell

Personal Thoughts/Goals:

_____

_____

_____

_____

Day 204

Be Fruitful and Multiply

Then God blessed them and God said to them "Be fruitful and multiply..." (Genesis 1:28).

The Lord designed us in His image to multiply. People were placed on the earth to have dominion and to increase God's Kingdom. The stress associated with the "rat race" of life depletes our body of nutrients required for restoration and the continuation of being fruitful. I have recommended drugless protocols for couples not capable of creating life and have seen children born full term as a result.

Pregnancy is not always easily possible for individuals with low thyroid gland function. I commonly suggest whole food, organic iodine, and/or kelp (a source of iodine) to fulfill the need for this required thyroid nutrient. The adrenal gland (a walnut-size tissue located on top of the kidneys) is a source of another important factor—progesterone. Progesterone is often deficient in individuals who are not capable of carrying a child full term. Also, the antinutrient—*sugar*—sabotages the body from properly carrying out its desire to reproduce itself.

Natural Prescription for Health: Add organic kelp tablets, deep ocean fish, and alfalfa sprouts or tablets to feed the thyroid iodine.

Personal Thoughts/Goals:

_____

_____

_____

_____

Day 205

"Wait Until You Have Weaned Him"

…Then the woman stayed and nursed her son until she had weaned him (1 Samuel 1:23).

There are natural laws and principles that do not change. God designed females' breasts to feed their offspring. Human breast milk has the factors in it to promote a strong immune system. Children who are bottle fed with human-made formulas often have allergies. Soy-based formulas can deplete the body of zinc and calcium. Girls who were raised on baby formula may have accelerated menses.

I encourage my patients to prepare for breast feeding by applying lanolin to their breasts prior to delivery. This will enhance the integrity of the tissue where most suction and/or friction occurs. You should also obtain a breast pump. Human milk can be stored in a freezer for the days when you are not able to personally feed the infant. It would also be wise to attend a LaLeche meeting to learn the benefits and techniques of successful breast feeding.

Remember, Mom, what you eat is what the baby eats.

Natural Prescription for Health: Cow's milk is for cows! What did Jesus eat? (I see a new bracelet—WDJE!)

Personal Thoughts/Goals:

_____

_____

_____

_____

Day 206

Wrinkle Free

...Not having spot or wrinkle or any such thing, but she should be holy and without blemish (Ephesians 5:27).

Paul was using skin as a visual when speaking to the Ephesians about marriage. Billions of dollars are circulated every year to minimize the onset of the natural aging process. Wrinkles and blemishes on the skin are a sign of internal breakdown in the body. It is an inside out healing process.

Healing and restoration nature's way is an inside-out proposition. Cigarette smoking depletes the body of collagen and sulfur, both of which are significantly needed for a smooth baby face. Sulfur can be sourced naturally from eggs, onions, cabbage, and garlic. Zinc is necessary for wound healing. Large facial pores occur with zinc depletion.

Hydration is needed for smooth skin texture. Drink water from a pure filtered source. Kidney stress or congestion can lead to a backup that affects liver function. You need optimal liver function for vitamin A use, which is needed for skin repair. Vitamin A, easily obtained from raw organic carrots, helps attain and retain that baby-face glow. We also have success adding a quality-sourced Omega 3 fat either by liquid or capsule.

Natural Prescription for Health: Drink a minimum of one quart of purified water daily.

Personal Thoughts/Goals:

_____

_____

_____

_____

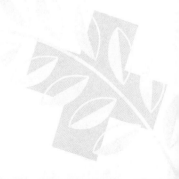

Day 207

Easily Bruised

The Lord will afflict you with the boils of Egypt and with tumors, scurvy [bruising], *and the itch, from which you cannot be cured* (Deuteronomy 28:27 NLT).

Often, Jesus would heal people in response to attacks by the Pharisees. He would heal them all.

Broken blood vessels result in blood escaping into tissue, leading to bruising. Bruising is not uncommon in women with heavy menstrual flow, and heavy menstrual flow generally occurs with high estrogen. Clean up your choices—no sugar, no trans fat.

A real issue today is that people do not eat vitamin C–rich food. One-third of all children and teenagers (four to nineteen years of age) in America eat fast-food meals daily.[36] Do you think they choose apples, pears, peppers, or kiwi? Vitamin C deficiencies result in poor collagen formation needed for blood vessel wall strength. You will bruise easily without a continued supply of vitamin C. Also, lack of vitamin C over time results in a condition called scurvy. By the way, oxygen quickly combines with the vitamin C in citrus, making it a poor source.

Aspirin use, which disrupts your body from working properly, creates fragile blood cells resulting in bruises. Use flax oil for pain and to keep blood cells moving freely.

Natural Prescription for Health: Have vitamin C–rich, colored bell peppers as a midmorning snack.

Personal Thoughts/Goals:

_____

_____

_____

_____

Day 208

Esther's Body Lotion

Each young woman's turn came to go in to King Ahasuerus after she had completed twelve months' preparation, according to the regulations for the women, for thus were the days of their preparation apportioned: six months with oil of myrrh, and six months with perfumes and preparations for beautifying women (Esther 2:12).

Esther was in preparation for twelve months before seeing King Ahasuerus. Oil of myrrh and perfumes were used for beatifying Esther. Today lotions and body applications may create a toxic state. Become a label reader. Sodium lauryl sulfate (SLS) and sodium laureth sulfate (SLES) are major ingredients in cosmetics, toothpaste, and ninety percent of all shampoos and products that foam. They have been described as "dangerous beauty." Studies on test animals using SLS or SLES show eye damage, depression, labored breathing, diarrhea, severe skin irritation, and corrosion. SLS, when combined with other chemicals, can be transformed into cancer-forming compounds.[37]

I want you to be aware of what you put *in and on* your body. What you apply is absorbed through the skin and travels through the lymphatic system and is processed in the liver. Look for beauty products *without* SLS and SLES.

Natural Prescription for Health: Read all labels of products that you apply to your skin. They may be causing chronic pain, allergies, skin irritations, and depression.

Personal Thoughts/Goals:

_____

_____

_____

_____

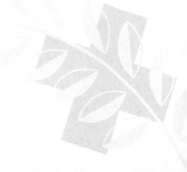

Day 209

Troubleshooting Belly Pain

And He said to them, "What kind of conversation is this that you have with one another as you walk and are sad? (Luke 24:17).

The godly insight alone from this tip will justify the time spent reading these daily nuggets. It is possible that, after *all* other logical causes of stomach pain have been ruled out, emotional sadness and distress may, in fact, be causing your pain.

Your diaphragm is a part of the emotional triad of health. The depth of your breathing is restricted when your diaphragm is not fully relaxing or contracting. The diaphragm shares an attachment with another muscle called the psoas, which is centered in the lower belly. When you have emotional sadness such as when your child begins kindergarten, leaves for college, or is first married, plus any other transition, you may experience pain, especially slightly off to the right upper quadrant. A skilled massage therapist can help relax the imbalance. I have had many smiling patients "high five" me after they had their diaphragm balanced. *Enjoy* these times of transition!

Natural Prescription for Health: You have earned a stress-relieving massage.

Personal Thoughts/Goals:

_____

_____

_____

_____

Day 210

Fatty Foods & Breast Cancer

Women who eat more animal fat have a higher risk of premenopausal breast cancer. (In earlier studies, the same researchers found no link to postmenopausal women.) For roughly eight years, researchers tracked the diets of more than 90,000 premenopausal women, 7,800 of whom were diagnosed with breast cancer (average age: forty-three) during that time. The risk of breast cancer was linked to red meat, whole milk, cream, ice cream, butter, cream cheese, and other cheeses (except cottage and ricotta).[38]

Natural Prescription for Health: Not all studies agree with these findings, though few have tracked so many premenopausal women. Nevertheless, it's worth cutting back on full-fat dairy foods and red meat to lower the risk of heart disease.

> When I first came to see Dr. DeMaria, I had irritable bowel syndrome combined with lower back and shoulder pain. I didn't take much medication for IBS, only a little occasionally for constipation or diarrhea. I didn't know how much IBS had weakened my body until I ended up in the emergency room about three years ago. The parasites in my colon had weakened my body. Dr. Bob recommended Parablast and that brought healing to my colon and the parasites vanished. I have also modified my diet per Dr. Bob's recommendation. I now eat more raw fruits and vegetables along with more fiber. I have also increased my water intake. I now exercise; speed walking for one hour approximately four to five days per week. Self-discipline has been the most difficult, making sure I'm releasing stress daily by getting enough exercise, eating a more balanced diet, and gaining spiritual strength by prayers and meditation. The adjustments have enhanced my health by diminishing colon pain, lower back pain, and shoulder pain. I have more energy and stamina, and my body feels more relaxed. —Janice Mokosh

Personal Thoughts/Goals:

_____

_____

_____

_____

Optimal Health for Men

Men need to spend time with their families. Plan time to be with your immediate family daily. Turn off the media and game center for twenty-one days and concentrate on your family. Start with a minimum of ten minutes daily for one week and then work up to thirty minutes—find one activity all can agree on. From Day 15 on, go for a walk together or ride or drive—look at the stars, read a book out loud to each other. I continue to have regular time with my sons and wife every day. Set up a time and commit to each other.

A common issue in men's health is a large abdomen. Men, I believe, eat too many carbohydrates, including alcohol or soda, which leads to the "pendulous" abdomen. Cut down on sweet snacks, take flax oil daily, and exercise with the family.

Men, we are living in a very serious hormonal health crisis at this moment in time. Gentleman, I am not sure if you are aware of the fact, but there are enormous levels of synthetic toxins vying to sabotage optimal levels of your potential *excellent* health; estrogen-based toxins are lurking everywhere, paralyzing a man's hormonal ability and the body's detoxification ability to function on all cylinders.

Women have the innate capacity to process natural estrogen; however, with the magnitude of xeno-hormone estrogens in our environment, even the God-given system designed to process estrogen has been burdened and compromised in females—hence women contend with heavy menses, breast cancer, cysts, and tumors.

We are currently being aggressively bombarded at all levels of media advertising under the banner of "Low T," that is small or minimal testosterone levels, which are the primary male hormone. I would never have thought I would be writing a tip in regard to the subject of low male hormones. It has been *suggested that up to thirty million American men do not have adequate levels of testosterone;* body signals of low testosterone include the following:

1. Emotional Passivity

2. Reduced Initiative

3. Enlarged Prostate and Breasts

4. Depression

5. Osteoporosis

6. Loss of Muscle Tone

7. Loss of Height

8. Frequent Nighttime Urination

9. Pain on the Inside of the Heels

10. Erectile Dysfunction

So what can be done with the challenge? First I would suggest you read, *Dr. Bob's Mens' Health—The Basics.* I have designed the book to be male-reader friendly with action steps.

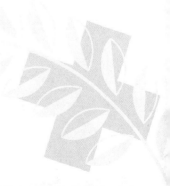

Day 211

Jacob's Hip

Now when He saw that he did not prevail against him, He touched the socket of his hip; and the socket of Jacob's hip was out of joint as He wrestled with him (Genesis 32:25).

Jacob was a fighter. He fought until the angel of the Lord knocked his hip out of joint. Hip alignment is one of the keys in carrying body weight. A posture imbalance, with weight being carried on one side more than the other because of trauma or injury, can cause one hip to wear out before the other. Obesity creates enormous additional stress for the hips. Smoking depletes the body of blood flow and minerals for cartilage strength. Groin pain, especially in males with pain radiating into the testicle area, creates a concern. I have helped many males about to have a testicle removed due to pain because of pelvic bone misalignment. A twisted pelvis from injury can be corrected naturally over time.

It is always wise to have more than one opinion from a variety of specialists before you submit to surgery. Have an appropriate assessment for hip and pelvis pain including standing postural X-rays. We weigh our patients with twin scales. You can do this with two bathroom scales, placing one foot on each scale. Do not look down, you will tilt the scale. Have someone else read the numbers on each scale.

Natural Prescription for Health: Look at heel wear on your shoes. Uneven wear may indicate pelvic hip imbalance.

Personal Thoughts/Goals:

_____

_____

_____

_____

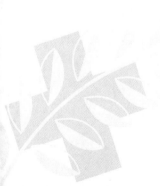

Day 212

Breathe Deep

And the Lord God formed man of the dust of the ground, and breathed into his nostrils the breath of life; and man became a living being (Genesis 2:7).

Oxygen is essential for life. God breathed life into Adam. It has been suggested that the air we breathe has less oxygen today than twenty years ago. The air cleaning product line appears to be limitless. Recycled air switches on the instrument panel of cars are now standard equipment.

Deep breathing belly exercises strengthen the abdominal tissues responsible for lung expansion. Taking a few deep breaths periodically is like giving your brain a blast of unexpected oxygen. Your neurons will celebrate. Try it, your brain will thank you. I also have suggested that patients breathe in through their nose and determine which nostril is not functioning at full capacity. Plug the one with the most intake and breathe in the nostril that was functioning less.

Also, erect postural alignment expands the lung's ability to take in more oxygen for fuel.

Natural Prescription for Health: Stand and take ten deep breaths.

Personal Thoughts/Goals:

_____

_____

_____

_____

Day 213

Mineral Tissue Analysis

...The hair on [Samson's] *head began to grow again...* (Judges 16:22).

Samson's strength from the Lord was a result of his being a Nazarite and not having a razor remove the hair on his head. Interesting. Today modern technology, with the analysis of minerals in hair, can reveal insightful information.

I commonly see a deficiency of zinc in individuals who have low energy. Zinc is needed to make insulin, a factor needed for carbohydrate metabolism. Copper is often elevated in individuals with a low zinc level. When copper is elevated in females, I also see high estrogen levels with associated symptoms of PMS—heavy menstrual flow and tender breast tissue.

Low zinc affects the male prostate. A deficiency can cause swelling. Memory loss can also be associated with low zinc. Are you tired? Do you have one of the PMS symptoms? Reduce wheat and soy as they deplete zinc. Raw pumpkin seeds are an excellent source of zinc.

Natural Prescription for Health: Hair mineral tissue analysis is a logical evaluation of body function.

Personal Thoughts/Goals:

_____

_____

_____

_____

Day 214

Do Not Fear

If the Lord delights in us, then He will bring us into this land and give it to us,
"a land which flows with milk and honey." Only do not rebel against the Lord, nor fear
the people of the land for they are our bread; their protection has departed from
them, and the Lord is with us. Do not fear them (Numbers 14:8-9).

Have you or a loved one recently received a doctor's report revealing bad news? Do not fear! I treat patients who have been given reports that are a wake-up call to change lifestyle patterns or face the consequences. You cannot expect different results if you continue to repeat the same daily harmful activity. Do not misunderstand me. I am not suggesting you ignore the report. I just finished a conversation with a female patient who had real long-term symptoms that did not respond to standard medication. She had been to several physicians without success. Her current physician suggested psychiatric care. I assessed her condition and made the appropriate spinal correction, which gave her an immediate positive response.

Other individuals may need to detoxify with colon irrigation and liver cleansing. A majority of the time, media-promoted healthy foods—including yogurt, peanuts, bananas, soy, and whole wheat bread—precipitate a constant reaction and body signals of pain. Typically what you crave is often the item that creates body symptoms and food sensitivity reactions.

Natural Prescription for Health: Think and pray. Study yourself. Seek multiple opinions. Common sense rules.

Personal Thoughts/Goals:

_____

_____

_____

_____

Day 215

Green Toes

They are all adulterers. Like an oven heated by a baker—he ceases stirring the fire after kneading the dough, until it is leavened (Hosea 7:4).

Yeast is used in baked goods and permeates with distinction.

Jesus took the time to wash His disciples' feet. This was a symbolic gesture of being a servant. Foot and toe health is a snapshot of whole body function. Pain on the inside of the heels *may* indicate prostate issues. When you have a full body yeast problem, it can result in fungus growth under all the nails. Fungus on the toes creates green coloration—this is serious.

Yeast and fungus grow in a sweet environment. We strongly encourage our patients to avoid baked goods with yeast, sweet fruits, and sugar. Full body yeast and fungus also may cause jockstrap itch in men. Focus on foods with low sugar, greens, and protein. Avoid fruit juices. We use a product called Agrisept, which is a citric seed extract derived from lemon, tangerine, and grapefruit seeds. This is not the same as citrus flesh. You can take the Agrisept internally and as a soak. Toenail fungus may take several months to resolve. Also try Epsom soaks with hot water to increase healing blood flow.

Natural Prescription for Health: Replace juice with hot water and lemon. Avoid baked goods.

Personal Thoughts/Goals:

_____

_____

_____

_____

Day 216

For Men Only—Who Wipes the Dish?

...I will wipe Jerusalem as one wipes a dish, wiping it and turning it upside down
(2 Kings 21:13).

Jesus came to be a servant and set us free. Men, I am setting some of you who need it free from cultural limitation and bondage. Here's the deal.

Do you thoroughly enjoy your life? If not, why not? Where do you put your socks? Do you iron the hanger wrinkles in your pants? Who prepares your breakfast, lunch, and dinner? (Obviously, single men, you do it yourself.)

Let's turn it up a notch! I am strongly encouraging you to develop and grow your servant's heart and mindset. I am speaking from forty years of dating and marriage experience of serving my wife and children.

Gentlemen, I would suggest that due to the law of reciprocity it would be to your benefit if you put your soiled clothes in the appropriate agreed-upon location; cleaned up shaven hair particles, dropped toothpaste, and debris in the sink and counter; washed and dried dishes and/or put them in the dishwasher and empty the dishwasher; and cleaned the lint filter in the dryer—all without complaining. Do not seek a "thank you."

Got it? Be blessed—*now move!*

Natural Prescription for Health: Look for domestic chores that need to be done in the house and do them.

Personal Thoughts/Goals:

_____

_____

_____

_____

Day 217

Don't Sit Still

It's not just exercise, but other movement (standing, walking, talking, fidgeting, and so forth) that keeps some people lean. For ten days, researchers tracked the posture and the movements made by ten lean and ten mildly obese people, all self-proclaimed "couch potatoes."

The results: the "big potatoes" stayed seated for about two and a half hours longer per day than the "small fries." That means the obese group burned about 350 fewer calories a day—a difference that translates into thirty-three pounds a year.

Alas, it's not so easy to change. For two months, the researchers put seven members of the obese group on a diet (they lost eighteen pounds) and obverted the lean folks (they gained nine pounds). Losing or gaining weight made no difference in how much either group moved, sat, or stood.[39]

Natural Prescription for Health: If you're overweight, keep moving. Walk rather than ride. Don't sit when you can stand, and keep moving when you have to sit. Move to the music from your car radio. Lift weights or do sit-ups while you watch TV, and so forth.

> Before making Dr. DeMaria's recommended lifestyle changes, I had yearly bronchitis and winter colds and felt sluggish a good bit of the time. I was on one medication. I changed my poor eating habits and now exercise. My attitude is now more optimistic, and I seem to be happier and more content. Overall I just feel much better with more energy. —Roger Hales

Personal Thoughts/Goals:

_____

_____

_____

_____

Day 218

Children Are a Reward From the Lord

Children are a gift from the Lord; they are a reward from Him (Psalm 127:3 NLT).

Children are an awesome responsibility. It is a privilege to bring children into the world, nurture them, and watch them blossom and fly. I have two sons that my wife, Deb, and I are extremely happy to have continue the next generation.

Do you want happy, healthy children? Speak happy, healthy, uplifting words. Do not make your children live your dreams. They have dreams of their own. I limit TV and monitor the computer and music they listen to. Know who their friends are and confront issues. We spent family time together on weekends with specific time of reflection and conversation. Take short trips together when you don't have the budget for longer vacations, such as weekend college football games, fishing outings, the zoo, ball games, museums, plays, musicals, high school events, or play soccer. There is a huge list of events to match all schedules and budgets.

Attending a worship service regularly will put God in the family. Attending Sunday School classes and being involved in a godly environment is an asset to strong family foundation principles.

Natural Prescription for Health: Looking at family pictures and videos/DVDs or your online stored memories are fun moments spent together.

Personal Thoughts/Goals:

_____

_____

_____

_____

Day 219

Upon This Rock

*I also say to you that you are Peter, and on this **rock** I will build My church…*
(Matthew 16:18, emphasis added). (Christ is the rock—the chief cornerstone.)

The geography in Israel corresponds to statements Jesus made in God's Word. When Jesus questioned Peter about who He was, the response of the Christ being the ro'' correlates with the huge cliff and rock formation in Caesarea-Philippi where Jesus and His disciples were when He spoke with Peter.

Assimilating rock minerals is necessary for proper body function. I have noticed, especially in men, a mineral consumption and absorption issue resulting in bowed legs. You need to have quality minerals for structures to support the body. Exposure to sun depletes the body of calcium. An excellent source of calcium includes (beside rock) sesame seeds and almonds. I encourage my patients to avoid sea sources of calcium and digestive aide calcium tablets. Alfalfa sprouts and Celtic Sea Salt are also great sources of minerals.

Natural Prescription for Health: Look in the mirror. What is the alignment and position of your legs? Straight or bowed?

Personal Thoughts/Goals:

_____

_____

_____

_____

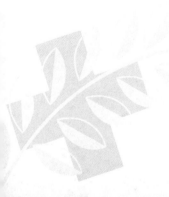

Day 220

Hair Loss

For every head shall be bald... (Jeremiah 48:37).

Body signals, including the number of hairs on your head (whether male or female) are windows to how the inside is functioning. A common cause of hair loss, especially seen in females, is a low thyroid. Additional common symptoms include cold hands and feet, headaches in the morning that diminish as the day goes on, constipation, fatigue, wide-spaced teeth, and thin, sparse hair.

In males I suggest a quality, organic flax oil—one tablespoon per one hundred pounds of body weight. Research in experimental testing suggests a deficiency in the Omega 3 fat, found in flax oil, creates baldness. Minerals are needed by the body to function optimally. We aid the thyroid by daily adding six to nine kelp tablets, a source of iodine.

I tend to see accelerated male pattern baldness in stressed males. Men, alfalfa tablets are an excellent source of minerals needed to keep hair on your head. Protein is also needed for quality hair.

Natural Prescription for Health: Take your armpit temperature for three days in the morning upon first arising. A temperature of 97.8 or below may suggest a need for organic iodine.

Personal Thoughts/Goals:

_____

_____

_____

_____

Day 221

Esau's Stew

*...Esau [Jacob's] brother came in from his hunting. Esau had also prepared savory food and brought it to his father and said to him, Let my father arise and eat of his son's **game**, that you may bless me* (Genesis 27:30 AMP, emphasis added).

The Bible is full of ideas for meals. Esau was a hunter. He served Isaac, his father, a special meal with the wild game he captured. My mouth is watering just thinking about the aroma, the essence of fresh herbs and venison he must have used. Preparing a blessing meal for a patriarch was a once-in-a-lifetime event.

When was the last time you had stew? Try making your next batch with a pressure cooker. Add some *new* vegetables. Live it up a little! Add some turnip, squash, and fresh herbs.

If you are a hunter and you consume wild game like venison, squirrel, or rabbit, here's a tip. Soak your meat in a citric seed extract to neutralize any "unfriendly" organisms. Cook your meat thoroughly. Parasites are easily transmitted in undercooked food. Wild game has the potential to have an abundance of parasites. This is one of several reasons why commercially prepared animals are treated with antibiotics.

Natural Prescription for Health: Do not microwave raw meat for a meal. *Never* microwave raw pork.

Personal Thoughts/Goals:

_____

_____

_____

_____

Day 222

Your Fuel Pump

*Then David and the people who were with him lifted up their voices and wept,
until they had **no more power** to weep* (1 Samuel 30:4, emphasis added).

Even a man of God can run out of gas. David and his men were exhausted when they
came to Ziklag. They were physically and emotionally drained. The adrenal gland
is your "Fight or Flight" escape backup—it is in a constant state of exhaustion for most
Westerners.

Does bright light bother your eyes? Do you wear sunglasses? Do you get dizzy
when you stand up from a sitting position? Crave salt? Always or easily fatigued? Take
cortisone? These are potential body signals that your body's fuel pump is tired. The
adrenal gland makes natural cortisone for pain relief, hormones for mineral absorption
preventing severe back pain, and hormones like progesterone and estrogen for sexual
function and a backup. The adrenals are fatigued from burning the candle at both ends
and eating refined carbohydrates such as cookies, cakes, pasta, and sweet fruits.

This is a very important gland that needs support to rebuild. We rehab our patients
with a specific adrenal protocol. The adrenal gland takes time to be reset. Reversing the
body signals mentioned above is a move in the right direction.

Natural Prescription for Health: Take time to rest between projects. The hours you
spend in bed sleeping before midnight are essential for optimal health.

Personal Thoughts/Goals:

_____

_____

_____

_____

Day 223

Cut Off My Headache

Therefore David ran and stood over the Philistine, took his sword and drew it out of its sheath and killed him, and cut of his head with it (1 Samuel 17:51).

David did a favor for Goliath by literally cutting off a headache. I am aware that you may figuratively like to have your head taken away sometimes. Headaches can be so painful that people have been known to pound their heads on a wall to relieve the head pain. I have treated many patients with that history.

Headaches that *don't* ever go away, regardless of treatment, need to be evaluated further with a head scan. Morning headaches that go away as the day progresses can be caused by a low functioning thyroid gland. Headaches at the base of the skull or top of the neck radiating to the top are commonly caused by tension with misalignment of upper neck vertebrae. This type responds to spinal corrective alignment. Work on eliminating the tension cause.

Challenging headaches include hormone fluctuation pain in females around the menstrual cycle. I normally see elevated estrogen levels in saliva testing suggesting inadequate liver clearing of estrogen, with not enough progesterone to cause equilibrium. This is best treated by consuming whole-grain B vitamin food, whole food B vitamin supplementation, and eliminating B vitamin-depleting sugar. Adding beets to the diet, along with flax oil (one tablespoon per one hundred pounds of body weight), is also recommended.

Natural Prescription for Health: To prevent morning headaches, do not eat fruit or sweets at night.

Personal Thoughts/Goals:

_____

_____

_____

_____

Day 224

The Beat Goes On

Taking fish oil supplements reduced the episodes of irregular heartbeats in a study of sixty-five people with cardiac arrhythmia. Patients who took enough fish oil (three grams a day) to supply one gram of Omega 3 fats had fewer arrhythmias over six months than similar patients who took three grams a day of olive oil.

Earlier studies had found a lower risk of sudden death heart attacks in people who eat more fish, presumably because Omega 3 fats stabilize the heart's rhythm. But researchers have only recently tested fish oil directly on people with arrhythmias.[40]

Natural Prescription for Health: If you have irregular heartbeats, ask your doctor if you should take fish supplements.

> The information that I have received from Dr. DeMaria has changed my life. I had been dealing with numbness in my legs and arms with unsteadiness and fatigue. I also have MS and take prescription Avonex for the MS. By changing my diet (no sugar, no dairy, eating healthier, and reducing stress) and taking the supplements suggested by Dr. Bob, along with subluxation correction, I feel one thousand percent better. I now have more energy. I don't feel poorly any longer, and this has led to a more positive mental outlook. Even with the MS, Dr. Bob has shown me how to work with my disorder and what is best for my situation in order to lead to a healthy, happy life. —Dave Page

Personal Thoughts/Goals:

_____

_____

_____

_____

Day 225

Slow to Anger

He who is slow to anger is better than the mighty, and he who rules
his spirit than he who takes a city (Proverbs 16:32).

Anger is an explosive emotion. Example: Road rage incidents are reported in epidemic proportions. We are blessed. The Lord knows we are dust and weak, and yet He is slow to anger.

Have you noticed the average commuter today? Besides talking on the phone while driving, people eat. The American kitchen table has been transferred to the vehicle. Gone are the days when the family sat down to breakfast, lunch, or dinner meals together. Games and events have clogged day planners and electronic calendars. Proverbs 15:17 reminds us, *"Better is a dinner of herbs where love is, than a fattened calf with hatred."*

We don't even eat real food on the run. Check out the ingredients of your favorite franchise. Foods consumed on the go—fries, soda, burgers—overwork the congested liver. An optimally functioning liver reduces anger when people are stressed. Anger requires the liver to work harder. Patients with emotional stress, including anger, tend to have more liver-related symptoms of disease including pain, gallbladder distress, arthritis, and even cancer.

Natural Prescription for Health: Make it a priority to eat in an environment of peace, often at home with loved ones.

Personal Thoughts/Goals:

_____

_____

_____

_____

Day 226

Gout

If the foot should say, "Because I am not a hand, I am not of the body,"
is it therefore not of the body? (1 Corinthians 12:15)

Gout is a common type of arthritis where there is too much uric acid in the blood, tissues, and urine. Uric acid is the end product of a food group called purines (pork and organ meats). The crystals can be sharp, which create pain, especially common in the big toe due to pressure in walking. Gout has been called the "rich man's disease" since it has been associated with too much rich food and alcohol. Pork and alcohol are common causes from my experience. *"Better is a little with the fear of the Lord, than great treasure with trouble. Better a dinner of herbs where love is, than a fatted calf with hatred"* (Prov. 15:16-17).

I encourage my patients to eat parsley with each meal. Parsley is a natural cleanser for kidney function. Men appear to have more "gout" attacks than women. From my experience, the kidneys kick in as the "second liver." When the liver is stressed, the overflow of toxins is placed on kidney function. Avoid pork, hot dogs, sausage, and alcohol. Clean machines work better.

Natural Prescription for Health: Turkey bacon makes a great BLT with safflower oil mayonnaise.

Personal Thoughts/Goals:

_____

_____

_____

_____

Day 227

The Mane of a Lion

The man [or woman] *whose hair has fallen from his head, he is bald, but he is clean*
(Leviticus 13:40).

Hair is a sign of authority and defines the gender. The mane of a lion, the beard on a man, and the hair on top of the head are significant. Hair loss in a short time period, either completely or partially, is a sign of internal stress. *Alopecia* is the term commonly used.

Your body requires additional minerals when stressed. Your body does not need hair on your head to survive. The minerals normally stored in the hair are used by the body as cellular spark plugs for chemical reactions to keep the engine going. The adrenal gland needs to be supported. Additional quality Omega 3 and 6 oils are required when you're under stress and experiencing quick hair loss. You need to determine the stressful source and address it, diminishing its emotional and physical effect. Supplement your diet with mineral-rich foods like alfalfa and Celtic Sea Salt. Avoid mineral-depleting sugar.

Natural Prescription for Health: Healthy fat from walnut pieces on your salad and Celtic Sea Salt add mineral spark plugs to your system.

Personal Thoughts/Goals:

_____

_____

_____

_____

Day 228

What Meat to Eat?

*He causes the **grass** to grow for the **cattle**, and the **vegetation** for the service of **man**...*
(Psalm 104:14, emphasis added).

What meat should you eat for optimal health? Should you eat meat and/or vegetables? What would Jesus do? God put cattle on the hills for a reason. There are benefits from eating red meat. My suggestion is to look for beef from an organic source. Antibiotics, growth hormones, and steroids are clipped onto the ears of cows in commercial farms. The additives enter the tissue of the coat and settle in highest concentration in fat.

Cows raised on grass (versus grain) on an open range where they can walk around have more health benefits. You can receive good fat from beef. I understand saturated fat has been associated with heart issues, but the right source of red meat, eaten in moderation, promotes life. You need protein made of amino acids for foundational growth. Red meat provides all the amino acids you need, plus vitamins and minerals. The source of meat and even vegetables available today has been modified by manufactures for a longer shelf life at the expense of health promotion properties. You want fresh and organic meat.

Natural Prescription for Health: Eat lean, grass fed, organic beef.

Personal Thoughts/Goals:

_____

_____

_____

_____

Day 229

Detective Work

*And it will become fine dust in all the land of Egypt, and it will cause **boils** that break out in sores on man and beast...* (Exodus 9:9, emphasis added).

The Egyptians were plagued with boils on their skin. Boils are a sign of potentially serious health concerns. Patients who present themselves to my office with a history of sores, open ulcers, and/or boils are instructed to have their blood sugar levels evaluated. One of the top devastating conditions affecting modern people is Type II diabetes. Boils erupt because bacteria thrive in a high blood sugar environment. Type II diabetes is accelerating in the number of new cases. It is estimated that current youngsters who are now two and three years old, will all potentially have a thirty percent rate to acquire Type II diabetes.

The significant point is that the condition is preventable. Just because a family member has a worn out pancreas does not mean you will. Change the recipe box of your diabetic relatives. Lose weight. This will take stress off the pancreas. Exercise will help use the glucose being circulated. Eating raw, whole food loaded with enzymes will take stress off the pancreas. Avoid processed food. Your body will have to work harder and wear out sooner with processed food.

Natural Prescription for Health: Have your blood glucose level evaluated if you have chronic infections and boils or sores that don't heal. I would request an A1C or also known as a HA1C if you suspect blood sugar stress.

Personal Thoughts/Goals:

_____

_____

_____

_____

Day 230

Magnetize Your Marriage

For this reason a man shall leave his father and mother and be joined to his wife…
(Genesis 2:24).

"*H*e *who finds a wife finds a good thing, and obtains favor from the Lord*" (Prov. 18:22). This proverb can go both ways. Poor health in females is due, in part, to bearing children and being stewards of the household. Men, help your spouses. Say proactive, life-enhancing comments *only,* or say nothing to your wife and family.

Both partners need to focus on serving the other without being recognized or thanked. Take the focus off of yourself. Increase your capacity to do more. Read God's Word with your spouse. Take a big step and pray together daily. My wife and I periodically take communion together at home in addition to our church service. Spend time with each other. Find someone to watch the kids, and create a romantic evening. Make a picnic lunch or go on a bicycle ride. Do you live by the beach, lake, or river? Water creates a calming background setting. To increase the attraction, let go of your agenda and fill the need of your mate.

Natural Prescription for Health: Focus on one day each month to magnetize your marriage.

Personal Thoughts/Goals:

_____

_____

_____

_____

Day 231

Gut Size and Gallstones

In a study of nearly thirty thousand men, those with at least a forty-inch waist had more than double the risk of developing gallstones compared to those with a waist measuring less than thirty-four inches. The risk was forty percent higher in men with a thirty-seven- or thirty-eight-inch waist and eighty percent higher in men with a thirty-nine-inch waist. Earlier studies had shown that being overweight also raises the risk of gallstones in women.[41]

In a second study, women who ate nuts at least five times a week had a twenty-five percent lower risk of gallbladder surgery than women who ate nuts less than once a month.[42]

Natural Prescription for Health: Roughly ten to twenty-five percent of US adults get gallstones.[43] If you're overweight, lose those excess pounds. Eating nuts may help lower the risk of gallstones, but nuts are calorie-dense, so don't overdo it.

When I first came to see Dr. DeMaria, I had arthritic pains in the knees and numbness in my hands. The medication that I had been prescribed created problems instead of eliminating the causes. I have appreciated Dr. Bob's honesty in evaluating that his care could not cure the problems, but he was certain that his care could improve the quality of life to existing limitations that existed. It has been difficult awaiting the improvements of my quality of living, but I am learning to address the causes instead of the symptom. My health is improving along with my quality of life. *Life* is one's willingness to help oneself instead of waiting for miracles. Living is making a living by what we get, but we make our life by what we are willing to give!
—Leonard Staysniak

Personal Thoughts/Goals:

_____

_____

_____

_____

Optimal Health for Children

Jesus learned by example from His parents. What you do is what your children will do. Talk to your children—avoid yelling. Read Bible stories to them regularly. Have a weekly or daily family time. Spend time with your children. Make life fun. Go to their events and cheer them on!

Create a loving, peaceful home environment. Children have real pain. Children love to be held and comforted.

Try cooking together on weekends. Always feed them food aimed at providing optimal health!

Day 232

Feed Your Kids Right

The children of your people will live in security. Their children's children will thrive in your presence (Psalm 102:28 NLT).

Children are precious, and what Grandma consumed, smoked, or drank has the potential to impact your child's health. I have observed that the second child often times can have liver congestion or stress because Mom and the first child—especially with the toxic food and pollution today—may have been overburdened. It is not uncommon for me to see female patients have their gallbladder removed after the second child due to an overworked liver from pregnancy.

What you feed your kids can overwork their livers, leading to liver stress even early in their lives. I have had eight-year-old patients who were told they needed gallbladder surgery. I really believe that breast feeding is best. Goat's milk is a viable option. Do not feed children solid food too soon. Avoid soda and hydrogenated fats. Watch the going-out-to-eat pattern. Avoid milk; it causes ear infections and allergies. Use almond, rice, or coconut milk. Soda pop depletes calcium, and the sodium benzoate can cause food allergies. Use almond butter for calcium. Purchase spelt flour bread, brown rice for a grain, and real oatmeal.

Natural Prescription for Health: Your children will eat what they see you eat. Eat healthy foods!

Personal Thoughts/Goals:

_____

_____

_____

_____

Day 233

Growing Pains

...They ate their food with gladness and simplicity of heart, praising God and having favor with all the people. And the Lord added to the church daily those who were being saved (Acts 2:46-47).

Israel migrated for forty years. Pain migrating in the body is really annoying for the adult patient and doubly painful for the parent of a child with growing pains in various parts of the body. My experience with adult patients is that pain that moves is associated with protein particles initiating a chemical reaction. For example, undigested protein particles from milk along with an inflamed intestine are primary precipitating factors.

Growing pains in children are commonly caused by a functional low thyroid. Cold hands and feet are a common low thyroid body signal. Measure a child's armpit temperature first thing in the morning *before* the child gets out of bed. The temperature should be 97.8 or above. I suggest organic iodine, one daily, if below 97.8 degrees. Vegetables, kelp, and Celtic Sea Salt are also sources of iodine. Flax oil and Omega 3 fat supports the intestinal lining and liver function for thyroid hormone and overall health.

Natural Prescription for Health: Add the above items, including sea vegetables, to the diet as a needed source of iodine.

Personal Thoughts/Goals:

_____

_____

_____

_____

Day 234

A Kor of Soda

The ordinance concerning oil, the bath of oil, is one-tenth of a bath from a kor.
A kor is a homer or ten baths, for ten baths are a homer (Ezekiel 45:14).

The average American consumes over a kor of soft drinks (soda) per year. A kor is a biblical measure of fifty-plus gallons. That's a lot of soda. Teenage males consume the most—as many as four to six twelve-ounce containers daily. Serving sizes continue to expand as do the waistlines of the more than fifteen to twenty percent obese youths in America. High fructose corn syrup, the primary sweetener, creates a cycle of endless thirst with calories added per gulp. Soda has an interesting preservative in the list of ingredients—sodium benzoate—that can create an environment promoting allergies. The phosphoric acid used for bubbles depletes the body of calcium. Attention: if you're taking medication for osteoporosis, you should know that the caramel coloring needs to be processed by the liver. Caramel, which is sourced from barley, also contributes gluten to the system. Notice the increased number of brown skin tabs on our youth. These markings are from liver stress.

Soda is not water and is not to be counted as a part of your daily water intake. Diet soda, regardless of your reason to drink it, causes enormous toxic stress to the liver.

Natural Prescription for Health: Spritzer sweetened with grape juice is a possible alternative for soda. Water rules as king of healthy beverages!

Personal Thoughts/Goals:

_____

_____

_____

_____

Day 235

Watch Your Company

Do not be deceived: "*Evil company corrupts good habits*" (1 Corinthians 15:33).

A challenge Paul dealt with while developing the early Church was mindsets. Once you have made a decision to alter your health lifestyle, seek out individuals with similar desires. Look at what people who didn't agree with Jesus did to Him. Jealousy, envy, and strife may occur because many may not like the changes you are making. This happens in my practice frequently. Let your light of improved health, weight loss, reduced pain, and emotional stability shine in the darkness.

People often resist change. Addiction to food and habits are perceived to be difficult to break. Individuals who crave milk may need fat, protein, and calcium. I tell patients to increase flax, chicken, turkey, beans, and sesame seeds. Sugar addictions are exceedingly common. We use a bile salt in protocols to remove fat from the available glucose so it is available. Chromium is a mineral that is often deficient in sugar cravings, which you may need to supplement into your diet. We add protein and use Agrisept, a citric seed extract, to control yeast, which causes a craving for sweets. Family members are commonly the most challenging. You can't change them; use your God-given discipline to say, "No thank you."

Natural Prescription for Health: Have alternatives to processed "goodies" on hand when you are confronted with a treat.

Personal Thoughts/Goals:

_____

_____

_____

_____

Day 236

What's Hot?

And standing over her, he rebuked the fever, and it left her; and immediately she got up...
(Luke 4:39 AMP).

Elevated body temperatures are not a disease but a symptom that may indicate the presence of disease. Having an elevated temperature is often helpful to the body. This is a defense mechanism of the body acting to destroy harmful microbes. A temperature above 102 degrees in adults or 103 degrees in children should be monitored by your healthcare provider. Logically fevers may be a problem for some such as cardiac patients or pregnant women. You should be checked by your healthcare provider if you have a headache, swollen glands, a rash, vomiting, or pain in the abdomen accompanied by a fever.

In my practice, especially for toddlers and children who are teething or in a growing mode, I see elevated normal temperatures stabilized by adding additional calcium supplementation to the diet. Calcium citrate or lactate are examples. Do not give a child aspirin to remedy a fever. Iron and zinc should also be avoided with a fever.

Natural Prescription for Health: Teething and bone growth require calcium. Childhood fevers often stabilize with calcium citrate or lactate.

Personal Thoughts/Goals:

_____

_____

_____

_____

Day 237

Children's Health

Blessed is the man who fears the Lord.... His descendants will be mighty on earth
(Psalm 112:1-2).

Be aware of what you feed your child's inside and apply to your child's outside. Baby oil is one hundred percent mineral oil. This substance is a commonly used petroleum ingredient that coats the skin just like what is used in plastic wrap. The skin's natural immune barrier is disrupted as this plastic coating inhibits its ability to breathe and absorb moisture and nutrition. The solvent prevents the skin's ability to release toxins because of the "plastic wrap," which can promote acne and other disorders. This process slows down skin function and normal cell development, causing the skin to prematurely age. I personally have assessed teenaged female patients with breast cysts that were associated with baby oil and observed oil droplets in the blood on phase contrast microscopy.

What you apply to your skin is easily absorbed through the lymph channels. Toxic accumulation occurs over time. Observe the number of brown marks on your teens. They increase in number as the liver is overloaded with fries, soda, and junk food.

Natural Prescription for Health: Read ingredient labels. What is applied to the skin—including self-tanner pigments and sprays—needs to be processed and incorporated into the cells or eliminated. Why overwork the system?

Personal Thoughts/Goals:

_____

_____

_____

_____

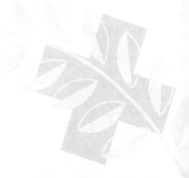

Day 238

Broken Bones and Colas

Active teenage girls who drink colas are more likely to break a bone than active girls who don't drink colas, says a study from the Harvard School of Public Health.

Grace Wyshak and colleagues asked 460 ninth- and tenth-grade girls about their history of broken bones, how active they were, and whether they drank carbonated beverages.

The 164 girls who were the most active were no more likely to drink colas than the others. But active girls who drank colas were five times more likely to have broken a bone than active girls who drank no cola. The link was much weaker for less active girls.

Why might colas weaken bones? "I believe it's the phosphoric acid in the colas, but we can't say with certainty," Wyshak reported.

The study has limitations, she acknowledges. It didn't measure bone density, didn't ask how much soda the girls drank, and isn't the kind of study that can prove cause-and-effect. Nevertheless, the results warrant further research.

"Adolescence is a critical time for bone development," said Wyshak. "How much bone you have when you're older is related to the peak bone mass you reach in adolescence." And less bone when you're older means a greater risk of osteoporosis.[44]

> I am in the sixth grade. When I first came to see Dr. Bob, I had back pain. I now do not eat as unhealthy as I did before. I loved sugar! It is hard sometimes to remember to eat better when I am with someone other than my mom. Since changing my junk food habits, along with the adjustments, my back pain does not happen as much anymore. It is virtually gone. Dr. Bob has been a big help to me and my mom. I'm glad my mom brought me to see him.
> —Logan Hinkle

Personal Thoughts/Goals:

_____

_____

_____

_____

Day 239

You Will Be Known by Your Fruit

For if the firstfruit is holy, the lump is also holy; and if the root is holy,
so are the branches (Romans 11:16).

The quality of fruit produced by a plant or tree is directly related to the health of the tree, the water, soil contents, and the sunshine or lack of it. The orchard attendant prunes, fertilizes, and scatters birds looking for food.

Your daily habit patterns create the state of the environment and fruit in your life. I treat many children who have behavioral and emotional issues that are categorized as Attention Deficit Hyperactivity Disorder (ADHD), Attention Deficit Disorder (ADD) or Hyperactivity. I have noticed a number of these children have parents with similar patterns. Sometimes I have to be firm with parents, helping them see that their choices and habits are mimicked by the fruit of their womb—their children. A common eating pattern is soda consumption. Soda is loaded with ingredients that stress the liver and nervous system. Sodium benzoate, which is used as a preservative, can be a cause of chronic allergies and ADHD or ADD. Grazing on partially hydrogenated snack foods impairs the body's ability to make essential brain fat. You may need to tend to your own garden more effectively.

Natural Prescription for Health: Spend time creating patterns that promote life for you and your family.

Personal Thoughts/Goals:

_____

_____

_____

_____

Day 240

Supersize Me!

Whoever keeps the law is a discerning son, but a companion of gluttons shames his father (Proverbs 28:7).

"Hold the pickle, hold the lettuce—special orders don't upset us." A familiar jingle. Another: "Two all-beef patties, special sauce, lettuce, cheese, pickles, onions on a sesame seed bun!" Is the fast food industry interested in your waistline? Hardly! Billions of dollars are made selling fast food every year. French fries alone account for nearly $20 billion of annual sales. Also, fountain drinks, which provide substantial income, promote obesity. Eating fast food over time can create liver disease and poor health. This is serious. The calories in the sandwiches are extremely high—up to one thousand calories per entree.

It is estimated that every day in America one-third of all youth between the ages of four and nineteen years eat at a fast food restaurant. And one- to two-year-old children who are healthy today have a statistical thirty percent chance of becoming a diabetic.[45]

What does all this mean to you? Develop new life patterns for you and your family. It is a matter of life and death. Plan your meals. Purchase an insulator bag with blue ice for travel. Almond butter and jelly travel well.

Natural Prescription for Health: Grate eggs with safflower oil mayonnaise and chives and roll in spelt or Ezekiel 4:9 pita bread (mostly found in health food stores).

Personal Thoughts/Goals:

_____

_____

_____

_____

Day 241

Cheek to Cheek

They gape at me with their mouth, they strike me reproachfully on the cheek
(Job 16:10).

" *If someone slaps you on one cheek, offer the other cheek also. If someone demands your coat, offer your shirt also*" (Luke 6:29 NLT). Injuring the cheek was a sign of great insult. What about modern internal insult?

Cheek health and integrity speak a book to an astute detective. Large facial pores are a sign of low zinc. Zinc can be depleted with wheat and soy consumption. Small blood vessels on the cheeks and nose may be a sign of elevated estrogen levels in females, suggesting a need for whole food B vitamins to process elevated estrogen levels. Small skin tabs and brown moles or nevi also suggest liver congestion. Eat grated raw or baked organic beets.

Small multiple "blackheads" suggest poor liver processing of fats and oils. Freckles showing up on the front cheeks by the nose bridge at about eight to twelve years old also suggest liver congestion with high copper and low zinc. Have the child eat an apple a day and take orange or cinnamon-flavored flax oil. Consuming dairy, especially for teens, congests the lymph system, resulting in facial acne. Finally, females with light, round patched bronzing on the *left* cheek nearly *always* have liver congestion and/or adrenal stress. This will go away over time, with appropriate diet changes, including no sugar.

Natural Prescription for Health: Substitute raw almonds and sesame seeds for calcium in teens with milk-induced acne.

Personal Thoughts/Goals:

_____

_____

_____

_____

Day 242

Spiritual Yeast

Therefore purge out the old leaven, that you may be a new lump, since you truly are unleavened. For indeed Christ, our Passover, was sacrificed for us...not with old leaven... of malice and wickedness, but with the unleavened bread of sincerity and truth
(1 Corinthians 5:7-8).

"Beware the leaven of the Pharisees," Jesus said to His disciples (see Matt. 16:11). Jesus was aware of the jealousy and envy in the hearts of the trained educated religious leaders of His time. Their deceitful hearts were compared to the yeast that raises the dough. Only a little leaven permeates an entire lump. Do not allow even a little into your life—or watch out.

A typical scenario goes like this. People like and eat sugar. Sugar paralyzes the immune system. White blood cells are impaired; bacteria and viruses can proliferate. This unchecked growth results in a system overload and breakdown. Your body attempts to fight off the bacteria and viruses, but because of the impaired white blood cell (WBC) activity, the unfriendly organisms multiply and win. You will experience symptoms like a cough, fever, lung congestion, and/or runny nose. Your first thought, *I need an antibiotic.* The conventional healthcare provider assesses you, writes a prescription, and all is over. Right? Wrong. Your body overcompensates with yeast overgrowth that has been allowed to hang out in your intestine without a balance since starting the antibiotics. Yeast release their own toxins into the system, and you feel lousy with mental fog, migrating joint pain, emotional distress, and so forth.

Natural Prescription for Health: Craving pizza and bread products may be a sign of yeast overgrowth.

Personal Thoughts/Goals:

_____

_____

_____

_____

Day 243

Upright Posture

…When [Saul] *stood among the people, he was taller than any of the people from his shoulders upward* (1 Samuel 10:23).

Gravity is a part of the curse. Lucifer fell out of Heaven. Falling involves gravity, which continuously and relentlessly pushes down on the planet. Even nature groans and is anxious about restoration to the Garden of Eden before the curse.

Maintaining erect posture requires energy. I instruct my patients to make a conscious effort to stand erect. Correct posture, with the shoulders gently rolled back, will increase the expansion of lung tissue (see figure). Increased chest capacity increases oxygen in the system promoting internal health with more energy, clearer thinking, and even reduced sickness.

An easy maneuver is to approach a doorjamb with your arms and hands at shoulder height. Lower your body into the doorjamb. Hold five seconds. The pull should be felt between the shoulders. Do three sets of fifteen daily.

Natural Prescription for Health: Focus on a conscious awareness to stand erect.

Personal Thoughts/Goals:

_____

_____

_____

_____

Day 244

Children

The righteous man walks in his integrity; his children are blessed after him
(Proverbs 20:7).

"*All your children shall be taught by the Lord, and great shall be the peace of your children*" (Isa. 54:13). We have two sons. We never talked "baby talk" to them. My wife breast fed them until they were twelve months old. The initial food we served them was mashed yams, mango, brown rice, and bananas. They did not drink dairy products. We spent our evenings reading and playing. Every night we were on our knees praying. We read Bible stories and simple books. On Saturdays, I made a special breakfast or we went out. Sunday was church and grandparents day. We established a regular pattern every day. My sons always knew when dad was home. My oldest son informed me recently that he does not want his children to have handheld game toys—I don't wonder why.

Spend time together and share responsibilities. Men, help your wives with as many domestic chores as possible.

Natural Prescription for Health: Spend time with your family. You only have them for a short time. Plan an event today.

Personal Thoughts/Goals:

_____

_____

_____

_____

Day 245

Fast Food and Teens

Adolescent girls who frequently eat fast food may add pounds they don't want or need.

Researchers at the University of Washington asked 101 healthy girls (ages eight to twelve) to keep one-week diet records when they started the study and again when they were eleven to nineteen years old. Girls who reported eating fast food at least twice a week gained more weight than girls who ate fast food once a week or not at all.[46]

Natural Prescription for Health: Most fast food is calorie dense, but anyone can minimize the damage by replacing the fries, burgers, and shakes with salads, a fruit-and-yogurt parfait, or grilled chicken.

> I had just started high school when I began seeing Dr. Bob. I had severe lower back pain that made simple daily tasks such as typing my homework painful and difficult. I didn't take prescription medication, but occasionally I would use medications for "curing" pains caused by sugar. Following Doctor's advice, I reduced my sugar in my diet and eliminated soda consumption. Cutting down on sweets was probably the hardest change. The information and care provided by Dr. DeMaria has not only removed the pain but also helped guide me to a healthier and more joyous life! It's real, and it really works! It may be trite, but you'll be glad you did!!! —Kenny Birdsall

Personal Thoughts/Goals:

_____

_____

_____

_____

Day 246

ADHD/ADD/Hyperactivity

In the fear of the Lord, there is strong confidence [wisdom],
And His children will have a place of refuge (Proverbs 14:26).

The mind and its potential is a frontier only scratched by our comprehension. A dilemma today is behavioral and emotional stability of children, adults, and seniors. The physiology of this breakdown is similar—the improper metabolism of fat.

There are five million American children diagnosed with Attention Deficit Hyperactivity Disorder (ADHD). For three months, I studied participants in a pilot program. My research revealed that eliminating trans fat is the leading factor for reducing ADHD symptoms. Trans fat sabotages your body from making DHA, the long-chain fat needed for brain health. Unfortunately trans fat or partially hydrogenated fat is everywhere. Depression responds to the same supplement protocol as ADHD. Avoid trans fat, take one salmon capsule per night for eighteen nights. Add six whole food B vitamins daily. Take B6, 150 milligrams daily; alfalfa tablets, six daily for a multiple nutrient mineral source; and finally, one tablespoon of flax per one hundred pounds of body weight. You will see changes in eighteen days. Limit dairy and consume no sugar. See the Glycemic Foods chart (pages 171–174) for sugar alternatives, as well as *Dr. Bob's Guide to Stop ADHD in 18 Days.*

Natural Prescription for Health: Baked sweet potato fries with sugar free catsup is a safe deep fry alternative.

Personal Thoughts/Goals:

_____

_____

_____

_____

Day 247

Teach Your Children This!

You shall love the Lord your God with all your heart, with all your soul, and with all your strength. …You shall teach them diligently to your children, and shall talk of them when you sit in your house… (Deuteronomy 6:5,7).

Is God in your family's life? Do you speak about the blessings of the Lord in your life? Our family time included reading Bible stories to our children out loud, especially from the Book of Proverbs. We pray before each meal, a sincere prayer time. Attending church service on Sunday and during the week creates an atmosphere of godliness.

Do you play Christian music at home or in your vehicle? Music with lyrics or instrumentals set the tone for peace in the household. David played the harp for Saul. The distressing spirit was placed there by God because of disobedience.

I do not want to appear legalistic; however, God's Word specifically says in the New and Old Testaments to love the Lord.

Natural Prescription for Health: Speak loving comments in your meal prayer time and conversation with the children in your life.

Personal Thoughts/Goals:

_____

_____

_____

_____

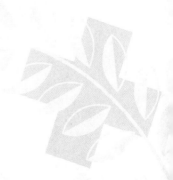

Day 248

Almond Butter

How is it you do not understand that I did not speak to you concerning bread?—but to beware of the leaven [yeast] *of the Pharisees and Sadducees* [peanuts] *(Matthew 16:11).*

Chronic health issues can have hidden causes that are commonly accepted. An example is peanut butter and jelly. PB&J is recognized by most as a staple Western meal—especially for children. My experience suggests that chronic sinus inflammation, allergies, headaches, and nasal congestion can be directly impacted by the amount of peanuts a person eats. Honey roasted are by far the biggest irritant. I have patients with long-term nasal passage health problems that completely disappear by eliminating peanut butter, peanuts, peanut candy, and edible peanut products. Peanuts have a mold or yeast as a part of their structure. This mold is toxic, especially over time with regular consumption.

Replace peanut butter with almond butter. Raw is best, but I use roasted and raw. Almonds are a quality source of calcium and are neutral in pH, being neither acid nor alkaline. To this point, I have not had a patient with a reaction to almonds.

Natural Prescription for Health: Sliced almonds add flavor to any stir-fry meal.

Personal Thoughts/Goals:

_____

_____

_____

_____

Day 249

Without a Blemish

Your lamb shall be without blemish… (Exodus 12:5).

God is not to be fooled or mocked. Our offerings and sacrifices are to be the best of our flock. As the temple of the Holy Spirit, we are to be without spiritual blemishes. How can you reduce physical blemishes and skin eruptions? What about the ones that seem to appear without cause on the left cheek? I have been blessed to learn that chronic left cheek blemishes are precipitated by liver congestion and adrenal gland stress. Why left? Liver and pancreas stress nearly always refer to the left neck, shoulder, and face, resulting in various signs and symptoms.

Cleaning up your diet by minimizing sugar alone will reduce the blemishes by thirty to forty percent in three months or less. It may take longer, depending on your state of toxicity. Blemishes all over your body equate to more *congestion* and work for you to do. Eat carrots on your salad daily. They are an excellent source of vitamin A. Your body uses vitamin A for skin and liver restoration.

Be patient. Do not have laser surgery for removing left cheek blemishes. They will return unless you clean your body from the inside out. I personally have witnessed many personal testimonies of whole body skin restoration. Always remember that skin is used as a part of the body detox system.

Natural Prescription for Health: Eat six baby carrots at your mid-afternoon break.

Personal Thoughts/Goals:

_____

_____

_____

_____

Day 250

Open Wide

He has broken my teeth with gravel... (Lamentations 3:16).

Jesus talked about the eye as an entrance to your spirit. I believe that the mouth is the entrance to your physical self. The integrity of teeth reveals much about the rest of the body. The position, color, alignment, and number of teeth affect your physical and emotional health.

Coffee and tobacco use can stain those pearly whites. The profit-driven market encourages us to use "teeth whiteners." However, low thyroid function can result in yellow teeth. Wide spaces between the front teeth may be the result of a thyroid that isn't working up to par. Soda consumption can create a phosphorous-calcium imbalance resulting in cavities when phosphorous is high or tartar when calcium is high. Loose teeth and a "pink toothbrush" can be a sign that more vitamin C from fruits and vegetables is required.

Brush regularly and floss the teeth you want to keep—all of them!

Natural Prescription for Health: Limit, then eliminate, soda use. The phosphoric acid (substance that creates bubbles) depletes calcium.

Personal Thoughts/Goals:

_____

_____

_____

_____

Day 251

Teach Your Kids Right

Train up a child in the way he should go, and when he is old he will not depart from it
(Proverbs 22:6).

"*A nd the Child* [Jesus] *grew and became strong in spirit, filled with wisdom; and the grace of God was upon him*" (Luke 2:40). How were you trained? What are you speaking into your children? Monkey see—monkey do. Spend time with your family. Children yearn to be with Mom and Dad. I have learned from experience that you need to place your children in an environment in which you wish for them to blossom and grow. I have two brothers. We were not allowed to watch the "Three Stooges" as children, which was a smart move on my parents' part.

What do you eat? Are you overweight? Children will pick up your habits. Children of parents who smoke have access to cigarettes. The same is true of alcohol, pornography, and drugs. The rich young ruler in Mark 10:20 answered and said to Him, "*Teacher, all these things I have kept from my youth.*" He loved money and possessions so much he missed a blessing. Children mirror their environment.

Natural Prescription for Health: Make an effort to spend quality time with your children.

Personal Thoughts/Goals:

_____

_____

_____

_____

313

Day 252

Peanut Allergy and Soy

A study in the *New England Journal of Medicine* reported that British preschool children were more likely to be allergic to peanuts if they had been fed soy milk or formula, had eczema or other rashes, were exposed to skin lotions with peanut oil, or had a family history of peanut allergy.

Soy protein could cause a cross-reaction to peanut protein, which has a similar chemical structure, the authors speculated. And it's possible that babies become sensitized to low levels of protein in peanut oil when it passes through inflamed skin.[47]

Natural Prescription for Health: It's too early to say whether soy milk or formula contributes to peanut allergies. To play it safe, avoid treating diaper rash, eczema, or other rashes with skin lotions that contain peanut oil.

> When I first brought my son to see Dr. DeMaria, he was overweight. I modified my son's eating habits, such as sugar intake, especially eliminating soda pop and adding more water. We also began an exercise program into his daily routine. The most difficult adjustment was modifying his sugar intake. The information we receive here is priceless. Our health and vitality has greatly improved, and as we stick to what we are taught, we do not get sick like so many people during the wintertime. By applying the wealth of info given here at this office, you get the results and also the quality of information that is given out of the passion and compassion to see people well—which is greatly appreciated and something that many people pay a lot of money for. We are so grateful! —Paul Schultz

Personal Thoughts/Goals:

_____

_____

_____

_____

Warranty Work

Clean machines work better. Water is the simplest, most cost-effective way to clean the body from the inside out. A suggestion during the next twenty-one days is to read the Book of Daniel and focus on what he did.

Do you need a breakthrough in your life? For twenty-one days focus on eating fruits and veggies only. Be creative. Eat squash, steamed veggies, and fruit. Avoid coffee, tea, and soda. This is an excellent semiannual protocol.

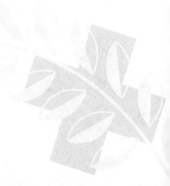

Day 253

Natural Healing

"So he went to him and bandaged his wounds, pouring on oil and wine..." (Luke 10:34).

Does it seem like you are always sick? Do your health challenges linger? Why do some people get colds, bronchitis, and the flu and others do not?

In my practice, I listen to what patients say, and it appears to me that unhappy and stressed employees are typically absent from their jobs. I have read that a large percentage of workers absolutely do not enjoy what they are doing. You have my permission to change.

Stress depletes an important nutrient required for healing of wounds and colds. Zinc deficiencies can slow your body's ability to repair itself. Meat is an excellent source of zinc; pumpkin seeds and alfalfa are good plant sources of zinc. Zinc is also depleted by wheat and soy consumption. Wound healing can be impaired by poor circulation, especially in the legs. We encourage chlorophyll ointment on wounds that are not responding to other methods. A body that heals slowly needs to be fed whole foods and detoxified of processed products.

Natural Prescription for Health: Add raw pumpkin seeds to your lunch salad.

Personal Thoughts/Goals:

_____

_____

_____

_____

Day 254

The Finest of Wheat

"He would have fed them…the finest of wheat…" (Psalm 81:16).

Our Heavenly Father always wants His children to have the best. Wheat is an excellent source of B vitamins and vitamin E. The challenge today is that wheat has been stripped of all its nutrients. White bread without the bran and outer coverings is nutritionally a poor staple in comparison to biblical bread.

I also see patients today, regardless of the source of wheat, who have some of their health issues caused by wheat sensitivities. I suggest that people should minimize wheat if they have chronic pain. Snoring may go away by eliminating wheat. Some food allergies are minimized by deleting wheat from your diet.

If you choose to eat wheat, I suggest whole wheat bread. Put olive oil or a pat of butter on your bread. Wheat sensitivities can be minimized by using olive oil and vitamin B6.

Natural Prescription for Health: Chronic allergies in your daily routine? Look for low gluten or gluten-free alternative grains—rice, spelt, and corn.

Personal Thoughts/Goals:

_____

_____

_____

_____

Day 255

Golgotha Hill

And they brought Him to the place Golgotha, which is translated, Place of a Skull
(Mark 15:22).

I was blessed to visit Israel and to be where Jesus was—walk where He walked. My preconceived idea of what I would see was based on artists' paintings and photographs taken long before urbanization. In reality, there is a massive bus station adjacent to the location where the crucifixion occurred. The toxins from the diesel fuel were quite putrid.

We live in a time when air pollution is common worldwide. These toxins can congest the lymphatic system and the liver. Continuous breathing of petrochemicals is also challenging for the lungs and kidneys. We use the herb "larch gum" to cleanse the lymph system. Parsley in hot water or salads supports kidney function. Snip dandelion leaves for your salad to stimulate liver cleaning; and goldenseal used in limited amounts accelerates lung cleansing.

Jesus came to die for our sin. He set us free from bondage. Set yourself free from the devastation of toxins. Keep your insides clean.

Natural Prescription for Health: Dandelion, goldenseal, fenugreek, and larch gum are all excellent God-given herbs for cleansing.

Personal Thoughts/Goals:

_____

_____

_____

_____

Day 256

Promoting Knee Strength

*Your words have upheld him who was stumbling, and you
have strengthened the feeble knees* (Job 4:4).

Knee pain, like pain anywhere, can be annoying. You need your knees to move. Here are a couple of thoughts from my experience helping those "achy knees."

Nagging pain on the inside of the knee can be from decay. Pain on the outside of the knee may oftentimes, ruling out an injury with an X-ray or MRI, be caused by gallbladder distress. Yes, you read right! There is a Chinese acupuncture point associated with the gallbladder on the outside of the right knee.

Eat baked or raw beets. Beets help purify the liver and gallbladder partnership. Eighty percent of knee strength comes from muscles on the front of the thigh. I have patients stand and squeeze the thigh muscles for a five-count up to three minutes daily. This will help most of you. Try it!

Natural Prescription for Health: Squeezing the muscle in the front of the thigh for a five-count, twenty times daily, will strengthen your knee and reduce pain by eighty percent.

Personal Thoughts/Goals:

_____

_____

_____

_____

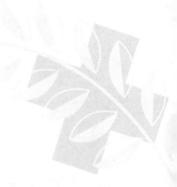

Day 257

Read My Lips

...An abomination to my lips (Proverbs 8:7).

Every part of the body has a significant connection to every other part of the human machine. Cracks at the corner of the mouth, where the lips connect, are commonly caused by a deficiency of a whole food B vitamin called Riboflavin. A thin upper lip is also precipitated by a B vitamin deficiency. Cold sore eruptions, from my evidence-based experience, nearly always point to a deficiency of easily assimilated calcium. I often see travelers returning from a "sunshine" vacation erupt with cold sores due to the fact that sunshine depletes the body's reserves of calcium. Stress-related issues have a devastating toll on the body's use of calcium.

Drinking water from a pure source bathes all the cells of the body including the lips.

Natural Prescription for Health: Add extra calcium citrate or lactate when you are spending long periods of time in the sun. Sea-sourced and digestive-aid-based calciums are challenging to absorb.

Personal Thoughts/Goals:

_____

_____

_____

_____

Day 258

Cruciferous Vegetables

He causes the grass to grow for the cattle, and vegetation for the service of man
(Psalm 104:14).

Broccoli, brussels sprouts, cabbage, and cauliflower fed to animals decreases cancer rates. Broccoli came to the United States in the early 1900s from Italy. The fiber from this food group assists the body in the elimination and binding of estrogen, reducing the risk for breast and ovarian cancer. Research suggests that there are protective agents found in these foods to prevent degenerative breakdown. Let food be your medicine. Chew everything thoroughly—and enjoy new levels of optimal health. You can also facilitate bowel movements by adding this additional fiber.

If you choose to eat peanuts, I would make sure that one of the cruciferous foods is included in your diet to act as an antidote to the aflatoxin found in peanuts. Patients who have a low functioning thyroid should limit cruciferous vegetables until thyroid function is improved.

Natural Prescription for Health: Rotate broccoli or cauliflower into your snack, salad, or supper regularly; rotate how you prepare the food items—raw, steamed, or sautéed.

Personal Thoughts/Goals:

_____

_____

_____

_____

Day 259

The Down-With-Diabetes Diet

Nothing can ward off diabetes like exercise and losing excess weight. But the foods you choose can also increase your risk.

In a study reported in the *Annals of Internal Medicine* (136: 201, 2002) of forty-two thousand men, the more "Western" their diet (red meat, processed meat, French fries, high-fat dairy products, refined grains, sweets, and desserts), the higher their risk of suffering from diabetes. A "prudent" diet (high in vegetables, fruit, fish, poultry, and whole grains) was not linked to a higher risk.

What to do: Eating a "prudent" diet should also cut your risk of heart disease, stroke, and some cancers. How convenient!

> I was bedridden or in a wheelchair for one and a half years due to a sporadic control of various muscles throughout my body. I was very foggy and unable to think clearly most of the time. Prior to being in a wheelchair, I took ibuprofen and allergy medications regularly. Also, antibiotics and anti-inflammatory drugs were taken frequently. I had also been on steroids, antidepressants, and something for autoimmune disease. The care and information from Dr. DeMaria saved my life! I believe I was on the path for far worse than a wheelchair had I not gone to his office.

> I had to modify everything. I received subluxation corrective care, whole food supplements, completely changed my diet, along with regular massages and colonics. I limited my schedule and commitments and even the way I handled and dealt with stress. I can't say that these changes were difficult because they were necessary. The alternative choice was to be in a wheelchair again and to not be able to think clearly. This motivator is what kept me going forward. The hardest change now is my time commitments. As I feel better, I want to do more, and I have to be careful not to fall into that trap again.

> I just want to say that prior to being in a wheelchair, I thought I was a normal individual with a hectic lifestyle and not so healthy eating habits, but nothing extremely bad. I had no idea that what I was doing to my body on the inside over all those years until my body gave up on me. Don't wait until your body gives up. Change your lifestyle before that happens! —Cindy Bublenic

Personal Thoughts/Goals:

_____

_____

_____

_____

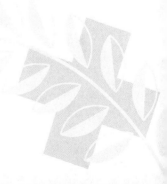

Day 260

Thoughts

Commit your works to the Lord, and your thoughts will be established (Proverbs 16:3).

The Lord knows the battlefield is in the mind. He is there, a lighthouse, a beacon, a focal point of rest. Thoughts race through our minds at limitless speed. A true dilemma in patients is the thought of impending doom or paranoia. Do you feel someone is looking over your shoulder? Do you cry without reason? Crying like this is typically a body signal of whole food B vitamin efficiencies. Relentless stress, which is common, depletes the body of B vitamins. You actually feel like you have raw nerves. The B vitamins are necessary ingredients for DNA, a protein needed for brain health and emotional function.

Thoughts, positive or negative, are a part of our existence. The ability to capture and control your emotional roller coaster and level it out will be enhanced by eliminating the major source of B vitamin depletion—sugar. The average American consumes in excess of 150 pounds of sugar per year. Sugar has the ability to paralyze your emotions and causes huge fluctuations in blood glucose levels. Sugar addiction can be controlled with minerals (chromium and protein).

Natural Prescription for Health: Look for whole food sugar alternatives. Avoid synthetic varieties—read labels. Pure stevia is a wiser choice than a product with maltodextrin.

Personal Thoughts/Goals:

_____

_____

_____

_____

Day 261

Good Ground

"But other seed fell on good ground and yielded a crop that sprang up, increased and produced: some thirtyfold, some sixty, and some a hundred." And He said to them "He who has ears to hear, let him hear!" (Mark 4:8-9).

Jesus was so simple in His teachings. Seed will flourish and multiply in good ground (see Mark 4:8). It is easy to understand; quality produce will come from good soil. Humanity was created by God from the dust of the ground (see Gen. 2:7). We, therefore, are physically made from dirt. You can survey the dirt in your body by evaluating mineral hair tissue analysis levels. Technology has created a venue to assist past and future potential patterns by comparing deficiencies and elevated mineral amounts.

Generally, I see low sodium and potassium in people with fatigue and sugar stress. Zinc levels are low and copper is high in women with elevated estrogen and sluggish liver/gallbladder activity. Selenium is low with a need for whole food vitamin E. Phosphorous is affected by protein breakdown. Toxic levels of aluminum and mercury are common with sluggish adrenal gland function. Calcium and magnesium are altered with thyroid function.

Eating food sourced from mineral rich organic soil is tastier and healthier than food from the over-farmed, pesticide- and herbicide-permeated conventional method.

Natural Prescription for Health: Mineral hair tissue analysis is a logical procedure to survey current levels of your "dirt."

Personal Thoughts/Goals:

_____

_____

_____

_____

Day 262

Ruddy, Fair Complexion

...David had a healthy reddish complexion and beautiful eyes, and was fine-looking...
(1 Samuel 16:12 AMP).

The skin comprises one of the largest organ systems in the body.

As a result of completing patients' mineral tissue hair analysis, I commonly observe a high level of copper in the hair of patients with fair complexion and "freckles." It is as if the copper is literally depositing in the skin. What causes the excess copper? There are a variety of possibilities, such as consistently consuming wheat and soy. This depletes the body of zinc with a resultant elevation of copper. Zinc is needed to make insulin, which is required for energy. Patients with low zinc are normally tired. Copper also congests the liver, which thickens bile. I have treated more gallbladder distress in individuals with fair complexions.

Beauty is only skin deep. God knew that the character of a person is in the person's heart. Samuel was learning a lesson in life when he anointed "ruddy" David with his fair complexion.

Natural Prescription for Health: Freckles are often associated with elevated copper and low zinc levels on mineral hair tissue analysis.

Personal Thoughts/Goals:

_____

_____

_____

_____

Day 263

Posture Weight Training

You shall have a perfect and just weight, a perfect and just measure, that your days may be lengthened in the land which the Lord your God is giving you (Deuteronomy 25:15).

The rules of nature are based on the survival of the fittest. Gravity continuously and relentlessly pushes down on top of us. It is not uncommon for me to have someone come to my office two or three inches shorter than what they were less than ten years prior. I see this in both men and women. Why?

Often the spine starts to break down because the muscles and ligaments supporting it are becoming weak and not toned to do their job. Weight training to tone muscle tissues only takes a few minutes, two or three times a week. I strongly suggest to all of my patients to obtain a large colored ball that you can fill with air. Lay on your back on the ball three to five minutes daily. Most sporting goods stores have light handheld weights. Hold the appropriate weight (three to twelve pounds) with both hands while laying on the ball; your arms should be above your head. Lower the arms slightly with elbows locked. This exercise will improve your posture, restore lost inches, and increase breathing capacity.

Natural Prescription for Health: Lay on your exercise ball five minutes daily.

Personal Thoughts/Goals:

_____

_____

_____

_____

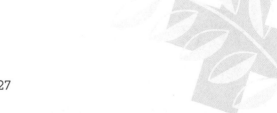

Day 264

Memory Boosters

Are not five sparrows sold for two copper coins?
And not one of them is forgotten before God (Luke 12:6).

God does not forget anything. Besides time, I believe your memory is your most precious health asset. What if you forgot crucial details such as: Did I go to the restroom? Did I have breakfast? When was the last time I bathed? Or how about the little important ones such as, "Where did I put my keys or glasses?" Alzheimer's and dementia are common today. Why? I believe the reasons include diet, stress, and bad effects from medication.

The leading culprit is the depletion of key vitamins and minerals by consuming too much sugar. Your body needs minerals and vitamins to make a brain fat called DHA. I see elevated aluminum levels in hair analysis testing with sugar eaters and patients with adrenal gland stress. Adrenal stress stagnates toxic mineral removal.

Keep your mind active with activities such as crossword puzzles and Scrabble. You need to exercise your mind like any other body tissue. Study and memorize Bible verses. We encourage flax oil, whole food B vitamins, and mixed greens for magnesium.

Natural Prescription for Health: Keep mineral levels high, Celtic Sea Salt, greens and seeds are excellent mineral sources.

Personal Thoughts/Goals:

_____

_____

_____

_____

Day 265

What Causes Your Teeth to Grind?

My flesh is caked with worms… (Job 7:5).

The devil is described as a lowly worm. Once settled in the body, the worm, especially a parasite, is very challenging. First you must recognize and detect it, then you must destroy and eliminate it. In my experience helping patients, this is one of the most difficult issues for patients to comprehend. Parasites do live in us. We have good and bad bacteria as a part of our normal digestion. Consuming sugar creates an environment in which unfriendly parasites like to grow.

Whenever I have a patient who enters my office with a history of conditions with no known cause, I always suspect parasites. Parasites can live in you an entire lifetime—if the environment is right. The most common consistent body signal is grinding teeth, especially at night. If you have a mouth guard for grinding, you may want to be checked for parasites. A high white blood cell, called eosinophil, on a complete blood count is a place to start but does not confirm.

Here is a very significant fact. Pregnant women and individuals with compromised or weak immune systems should not handle cat litter. Cats transmit an organism called toxoplasmosis gandi that can lead to health problems in humans.

Natural Prescription for Health: If you grind your teeth, get checked for parasites.

Personal Thoughts/Goals:

_____

_____

_____

_____

Day 266

Crosswords and Alzheimer's

Reading newspapers or books, playing games like cards or checkers, doing crosswords or other puzzles, going to museums, watching television, or listening to the radio—those and other activities that stimulate the mind may cut the risk of Alzheimer's disease.

Researchers asked more than eight hundred Alzheimer's-free people aged sixty-five or older how often they participated in mentally challenging activities. Four years later, the people who had reported more mental activity were less likely to have the disease. Physical activity had no impact on risk.

What to do: This study (*Neurology* 59:1910, 2002) doesn't *prove* that crossword puzzles will ward off Alzheimer's disease. If Alzheimer's starts ten years before it is diagnosed, it is possible that the people who didn't read or do puzzles already had an early form of the disease that was too mild for the researchers to detect when the study began. But it doesn't hurt to keep your mind moving.

> My life has improved one hundred percent since receiving information and care from Dr. DeMaria. Previously I could not walk. I kept falling due to serious nerve damage on my spine. It has been difficult, but I have stopped consuming sugar. I prayed to the Lord to send help to me. He sent Dr. Bob and his beautiful crew. They are all so helpful. —Eleanor Chinenti

Personal Thoughts/Goals:

_____

_____

_____

_____

Day 267

Can You Pass This Test?

But this He said to test him, for He Himself knew what He would do (John 6:6).

Abraham was tested. Jesus was tested, and now it's your turn. This is a set of questions for you to see if ADHD is an issue in your life. This Adult Self-Report is intended for individuals who are age eighteen years or older. Check the box that best describes how you felt or conducted yourself over the past six months.

Add the number of checkmarks that appear in the darkly shaded area. Four or more checkmarks indicate that your symptoms may be consistent with Adult ADHD. It may be beneficial for you to talk with your healthcare provider about an evaluation.

This test is also available at www.DruglessDoctor.com. Tell a friend. Obtain my book *Dr. Bob's Guide to stop ADHD in 18 Days*. It will take you to the next level of healthy living.

Natural Prescription for Health: Read the Word daily and focus on memorizing Bible verses. Keep your brain active.

Personal Thoughts/Goals:

_____

_____

_____

_____

	Never	Rarely	Sometimes	Often	Very Often
1. How often do you have trouble wrapping up the final details of a project, once the challenging parts have been done?					
2. How often do you have difficulty getting things in order when you have to do a task that requires organization?					
3. How often do you have problems remembering appointments or obligations?					
4. When you have a task that requires a lot of thought, how often do you avoid or delay getting started?					
5. How often do you fidget or squirm with your hands or feet when you have to sit down for a long time?					
6. How often do you feel overly active and compelled to do things, like you were driven by a motor?					

Day 268

Activate Your Hearing

He who has an ear, let him hear what the Spirit says... (Revelation 3:22).

Ears are designed for hearing. Hearing God's Word and allowing it to settle in and permeate your spirit promotes life. Our Creator, in His infinite wisdom, knows that clean machines work better.

Your body's self-healing nature can use ear canals for a detoxification site. I generally see abundant ear wax in individuals with compromised digestion, elimination, and toxic eating habits. For instance, individuals who smoke generally have more accumulation of wax than nonsmokers.

Another example is dairy consumption. We have been advised by the Dairy Association to drink more milk, but this may not be the best advice.

Natural Prescription for Health: If you have chronic ear wax accumulation and consistently consume milk, try reducing your dairy for a season. Chronic ear infections in children are commonly caused by dairy-sourced items.

Personal Thoughts/Goals:

_____

_____

_____

_____

Day 269

Carpal Tunnel Pain

…And none of the mighty men have found the use of their hands (Psalm 76:5).

Did you ever wonder why "Rosie the Riveter" was without carpal tunnel pain? Case studies and research on carpal tunnel focuses on the more recent epidemic of this dilemma. Carpal tunnel siphons from the economy millions of dollars of work time loss and treatment costs every year.

Do you suffer with carpal tunnel syndrome (CTS)? Try eliminating soda, cookies, and dairy from your snack habit. Drink purified water and eat almonds and veggie sticks as an alternative. Adding pain relieving flax oil from an organic source—one tablespoon per one hundred pounds of body weight along with 150 milligrams of whole food vitamin B6 will promote healing of the inflamed tissues. CTS of both wrists may be precipitated by a misaligned or a decayed neck vertebra and disc.

Natural Prescription for Health: Add 150 milligrams of whole food B6-Niacinamide to your routine if you suffer with wrist pain. Avoid soda, sugar, and trans fat, partially hydrogenated and hydrogenated.

Personal Thoughts/Goals:

_____

_____

_____

_____

Day 270

Life Without Back Pain

Why is my pain perpetual and my wound incurable, which refuses to be healed?...
(Jeremiah 15:18).

In Luke 13:13, the woman with back pain for eighteen years must have done cartwheels after Jesus released the devil's grip on her. The term mechanical back pain, a very common term in the field of manipulative care, can be a little oversimplified. Back pain is one of the leading causes of work absenteeism. There are a lot of variables.

The mechanics, or motion, of the spine may not be exactly one hundred percent, and the patient can be without pain one day and in misery the next. Discomfort in the joints is impacted by the activity of sensory receptors under direct influence of food choices, stress, smoking, water intake, trauma, and mechanics. X-rays of the spine are best taken standing with gravity playing its part on alignment. You need to know the position of a small muscle-ligament attachment called the spinous processes. I usually see pain on the side of spinous process rotation. Normally I make a spinal correction to move the spinous back to the proper position—it may have twisted right, for example, and I move it back to the left. I only correct the weak side, not both. A skilled spinal adjustor will know how to do this. Correcting both sides is more for mobilization, still good, but is not for long-term correction.

Back pain for long duration caused by food sensitivities versus bone or joint injury miraculously disappears when you delete dairy and citrus and stop smoking cigarettes. Test me on this!

Natural Prescription for Health: Bend to the side opposite back pain ten times daily, holding for a five-count.

Personal Thoughts/Goals:

_____

_____

_____

_____

Day 271

Sticks and Stones Will Break My Bones

He guards all his bones; not one of them is broken (Psalm 34:20).

Did you ever break a bone? Fractures can be painful, especially the ones that you cannot support or cast, such as a tailbone or nose. Bones have a rich supply of blood vessels and nerve endings. Regardless of what you do, it takes time for bones to heal and replace themselves.

Taking aspirin will slow down fracture repair. If aspirin slows fracture repair, I am sure it slows or interferes with regular bone replacement. I would wonder if women with osteoporosis should take aspirin. Osteoporosis fracture prevention can be helped with flax oil. Flax oil helps restore hormone function and calcium absorption. People who smoke cigarettes have impaired healing time also.

What about calcium? By far sesame seeds are one of the best sources of calcium. I sprinkle sesame seeds on my salad. If you have diverticulosis, try sesame seed butter.

Natural Prescription for Health: Try 2000 milligrams of royal jelly daily along with 150 milligrams of niacinamide B6 daily to diminish the desire for the nicotine in cigarettes—a natural remedy to stop smoking. Nightshades including tomatoes, white potatoes, eggplant, and green peppers tend to be addictive because they are a source of nicotine.

Personal Thoughts/Goals:

_____

_____

_____

_____

Day 272

The Truth About Cholesterol

You will know the truth, and the truth will set you free (John 8:32 NIV).

Know: to perceive, understand, recognize, gain knowledge, recognition of truth by personal experience (Strong's #1097).

I *know* from experience that you can reduce cholesterol by up to forty percent without toxic medication. Cholesterol is one of the most misunderstood and media-manipulated topics of the last twenty-five years. Cholesterol is not good or bad but *necessary*. Think of cholesterol as a firefighter on the way to a fire or inflammation. LDL is the name of the fire truck that takes LDL cholesterol to the fire. HDL is the name of the fire truck that takes it back to the station. Elevated LDL cholesterol occurs with a fire. More fire, more LDL cholesterol. Medication to lower cholesterol literally sidetracks LDL from going to the fire (blood vessel). Here is the key question: *What causes the fire?* If you can prevent or stop the fire, your LDL cholesterol will *not* need to rise to go to the fire.

My clinical research reveals that sugar, trans fat, stress, dairy, and red meat elevate pain-producing prostaglandin 2 that causes the fire. Flax oil helps put the fire out. Trans fat or partially hydrogenated fat, which is designed to lower cholesterol, actually raises it. My suggestion to you—backed up by research—is that you can lower cholesterol by adding beet fiber to your diet. Sugar, dairy, and trans fat irritate blood vessels.

Natural Prescription for Health: Add raw or baked beets (not canned or pickled) to your daily diet, with a dash of flax or olive oil. Avoid sugar.

Personal Thoughts/Goals:

_____

_____

_____

_____

Day 273

The Fifty Percent Myth

Only half of all heart attacks are caused by known risk factors like smoking, high cholesterol, diabetes, and high blood pressure. Or so people say. It's not clear where that myth started, but two new studies show that it's flat-out wrong.

In a study reported in the *Journal of the American Medical Association* (290: 891, 898, 947, 2003), one team of researchers examined three studies that tracked more than 386,000 people for between twenty to thirty years. A second team analyzed data on more than 122,000 people in 145 clinical trials. The conclusion: Between eighty and ninety percent of patients who were eventually diagnosed with heart disease—and more than ninety-five percent of patients who died of heart disease—had at least one of the major risk factors listed above.

What to do: Don't smoke. Use diet, exercise, and (if necessary) drugs to keep your cholesterol, blood pressure, blood sugar, and weight at healthy levels.

> I had high cholesterol, especially high LDLs, a slumping posture, and didn't eat enough protein foods when I first came to see Dr. DeMaria. I took Niacin daily along with aspirin and garlic to try and control the high LDLs. Dr. Bob shared that I needed to reduce my carb intake and begin eating more protein (this was difficult for me since I was accustomed to eating mostly carbs). I began eating a lower carb diet and added protein, i.e., eggs and red meat.
> I love that I get to eat eggs again while my cholesterol stays low! —Pat Dobson

Personal Thoughts/Goals:

_____

_____

_____

_____

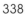

Body Building—From the Inside Out

Gravity continually and relentlessly compresses tissues. Daily postural supporting maneuvers are critical for proper digestion and breathing. You can slow the deterioration process by taking four or five minutes daily to stand erect. The head glide exercise (see Day 52) will relieve muscle tension in the neck. Go slowly; you may feel pain at first. Do this new pattern daily forever.

Internal mechanics are necessary for optimal health. There is a progression in the body where glands and organs can refer electrical impulses back to the area where the nerves innervating, or originally sending messages, are impacted. Let me give you a typical example that I see in the office and that is a real challenge for many people. The pancreas is a little known source of enzymes required for digestion and healthy function; fats require lipase, carbohydrates require amylase, and proteins need protease. A heavy load of dairy, for example, can stress the pancreas insidiously by pressing it to process the fat, carbs, and protein—this is a reason dairy products including yogurt, cottage cheese, and ice cream can be a cause of your mid-back and left neck pain. The left neck and mid-back region is the original development location of the pancreas, which eventually moved to its adult location in the mid-central abdomen. Referred glandular pain is a common cause of pain in nearly every patient I treat with chronic pain syndrome; it is inside out healing and building.

Anatomy

Adrenal Gland: A small walnut-shape gland located on top of the kidneys. The adrenal gland makes several hormones necessary for optimal health. It is important to make natural cortisone and male and female hormones, and it is critical for the maintenance of various minerals. The adrenal gland also creates the chemicals necessary for you to respond to emergencies. It is commonly weakened by sugar and stress. Chronic pain, female hormone issues, asthma, allergies plus so much more are directly affected by adrenal function. Two CD programs are available through our online resource library.

Gallbladder: A small reservoir located on the lower liver. It is necessary for optimal fat metabolism. The liver produces bile. I commonly see gallbladder issues in females with two or more children and men who eat processed fast food. Gallbladder removal requires a daily supplement of bile to assist processing of fat. The gallbladder does not grow back. If you have a history of gallbladder surgery, it is critical to change your diet. The pancreas works harder to process fat without the assistance of adequate bile from the liver with certain foods.

Liver: This is a body's work horse. It is located in the right lower rib cage. A damaged liver can be restored by making appropriate lifestyle changes, including limiting alcohol, sugar, and human-made chemicals. Diet soda is a leading cause of poor liver function. Toxic chemicals need to be processed by the liver. Skin lesions including acne and psoriasis will clear up. Female hormone issues, even tender breasts, heavy menstrual flow, and spider veins, will respond to liver cleansing. Eat organic beets regularly. Avoid lymph congesting, liver stressing, conventional, chemically-altered dairy products. CD programs are available online.

Lymph: The lymph system is the sewer system of the body. It also is one of the main defense or immune systems. Water and exercise are necessary for proper function. Dairy products slow the lymph movement. A proper functioning liver is needed for lymph clearing from the body.

Pancreas: The pancreas, we have been taught, is the organ that makes insulin necessary for glucose or blood sugar to get into cells. The pancreas also makes enzymes assisting in the metabolism of food. Enzymes are necessary for digestion and are commonly deficient because of processed food. Convenience food items have been robbed of most living cells to create a longer shelf life. Patients who eat sugar, dairy, and sweet fruits tend to have left neck and mid-back pain. I believe this is directly related to the pancreas embryologic development when we are in the womb. The pancreas refers pain to the left side primarily when it is overworked, much like an overworked motor shorts out a circuit. This is a common problem I see in my practice.

Thyroid Gland: The "gas pedal" of your body. The thyroid gland is located in the mid-throat region and is responsible for many functions including keeping you warm. This gland is commonly stressed by chlorine from showers and pools. It controls calcium and affects cholesterol levels. Common body signals of a weakened thyroid gland include: chronic constipation, thin hair, and morning headaches that wear off as the day progresses. You can monitor the function of your thyroid gland by monitoring your arm pit temperature first thing in the morning for ten minutes. The temperature normally should be 97.8 degrees. The thyroid responds to organic iodine and flax oil. The liver needs to be functioning optimally, assisting the body, to create thyroid hormone available for use. CD programs available online.

Day 274

As the Twig Is Bent—the Tree Will Grow

*You do not know what is the way of the wind, or how the bones grow
in the womb of her who is with child... (Ecclesiastes 11:5).*

Wind has the strength to shape trees. Besides Alzheimer's, one of the biggest concerns among individuals is acquiring the bent forward position, like Grandma developed when she aged. To improve posture and back strength, we use the Ball Exercise (see figure). I have had patients tell me that they literally grew two inches using this exercise.

Ball Exercise. Using a large exercise ball, lay with your back bent over the ball for three to five minutes daily. Start slowly.

Natural Prescription for Health: Measure your height before you start this maneuver. Expect to grow.

Personal Thoughts/Goals:

_____

_____

_____

_____

Day 275

"He Knows Our Frame"

For He knows our frame; He remembers that we are dust (Psalm 103:14).

God knows every detail of our construction. The human frame is an erect structure on two feet. Gravity continually pushes down on our bodies from head to toe.

The strength of your bony frame is critical for nervous system function. The spinal cord is in the column. You should focus on walking to strengthen your butt muscles; they extend your trunk and pelvis. Your lower back needs strong pelvic muscles for support.

The quality of food you consume effects bone structure. Heel spurs are common in patients who have an alkaline pH or consume baking soda. Our frame won't be balanced with heel spur pain.

Try "toe raises" to alleviate pain. While sitting in a stationary position with your feet straight forward and flat on the floor, raise your toes twenty-five times. Then turn your feet inward and repeat the toe raises twenty-five times. Turn your feet outward and repeat. This will strengthen foot structure, which supports the frame. Heel spur pain will go away over time. Make sure you minimize citrus food consumption. Use one tablespoon of organic apple cider vinegar daily on your mixed salad to help balance pH.

Natural Prescription for Health: Wear supportive shoes and take a brisk twenty- to thirty-minute walk with a friend. You can also stand on with one foot on the floor or stand on a foam Theraband™ stabilizer two to three minutes daily on each foot.

Personal Thoughts/Goals:

_____

_____

_____

_____

Day 276

Building Strong Bones

...And a good report makes the bones healthy (Proverbs 15:30).

Words have power. There is a part of the brain called the hypothalamus that connects the emotional and the physical person. It is your body's CEO. Paul, in Ephesians 5:19, said that we are to speak to each other in psalms and hymns. Paul knew that words have power.

When you are under emotional distress, your body uses more calcium to neutralize the acid environment caused by the negative emotions. That is why you will see cold sores or fever blisters on people who are having higher than normal negative emotional pressure. Your bones need calcium, protein, and other ingredients to be strong. A constant assault of negative circumstances and situations can deplete reserves of body calcium, including those found in bone matrix.

Watch what you say. Speak uplifting, positive statements. Speak God's Word in love.

Natural Prescription for Health: Kale, mixed greens, sesame seeds, walnuts, and almonds are an excellent source of minerals.

Personal Thoughts/Goals:

_____

_____

_____

_____

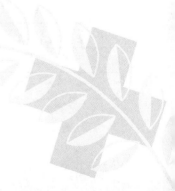

Day 277

Plantar Faciitis—Foot Pain

From the sole of the foot even to the head, there is no soundness in it,
but the wounds and bruises and putrefying sores; they have not been closed
or bound up, or soothed with ointment (Isaiah 1:6).

Feet are the foundation of our two-legged biped stance. Jesus talked about feet frequently. The feet of the people in Israel had no pain, and their sandals never wore out when walking in the desert for years. That's better than the high-priced sneakers of today.

One of the challenges for my patients is foot pain. Here's a hot tip for you. Burning feet are usually caused by poor or improper fat metabolism precipitated by a congested liver and a limited intake of vitamin B, including Choline and Inositol. Plantar Faciitis, which is pain along the tissue on the very bottom of the foot and heel area, is normally caused by not enough Omega 3 flax oil consumption, lack of vitamin B6, low thyroid, and weak adrenals. Thyroid function is needed for calcium absorption, which calms and relaxes tissues. The adrenals make natural cortisone.

A very light stretching exercise with mild resistance: Use an elastic band around the toes and with both hands pull the foot toward you. A few light stretches daily with additional flax oil, whole food B vitamin and B6, with kelp for iodine, which supports thyroid function, and whole vitamin C for adrenal support is a great start. Also, I suggest a little time off the feet. Wear an arch-support shoe versus flat or high-heeled shoes.

Natural Prescription for Health: Gently rubbing the bottom of your feet with pain-relieving castor oil is a great step to optimal foot health.

Personal Thoughts/Goals:

_____

_____

_____

_____

Day 278

Lessons Learned From Mummies

Now when they had departed, behold, an angel of the Lord appeared to Joseph in a dream, saying "Arise, take the young Child and his mother, flee to Egypt, and stay there until I bring you word..." (Matthew 2:13).

What did Jesus eat in Egypt? The chosen people had specific written guidelines for every aspect of their lives. God was protecting them from the environment at the time, including personal hygiene, toxic food choices, and daily life interactions. When Joseph, Mary, and Jesus were in Egypt, they adapted to a different culture. How do you think they were treated? The Egyptians knew they were once slaves. Meditate on that.

We have been blessed to learn from studying the remains of Egyptian mummies. They ate a diet much like we have been told to eat as of recently. Low fat, high carbohydrate, grains, and corn residue have been discovered in their stomachs upon dissection. Their blood vessels had scarring similar to individuals today who have high blood pressure.

"OK, Dr. Bob, what are you saying?" I am encouraging you to learn from the past. Increase flax oil consumption necessary to relieve pain and blood vessel inflammation. Minimize refined grains, and eat whole food, including raw, organic greens. The high carbohydrate diet increases insulin. Insulin will create retention of sodium and water, resulting in higher blood pressure. It is estimated only five percent of blood pressure cases are a result of salt intake.

Natural Prescription for Health: Monitor your blood pressure. Limit your pastry, cookie, pasta, and cake intake. Add flax and greens to your diet.

Personal Thoughts/Goals:

_____

_____

_____

_____

Day 279

She Was Bent Over

And He laid His hands on her, and immediately she was made straight, and glorified God
(Luke 13:13).

Can you even imagine being bent over for eighteen years? Jesus knew this woman had a spirit of infirmity.

Do you suffer with relentless spinal pain and discomfort? I have assessed patients with a lifetime of spinal discomfort. I always rule out spinal pathology, abnormal joints, and alignment. Appropriate spinal correction is applied, normally very successfully. I have had chronic cases when the patient is unaware of the cause of the pain. Do you know the most common causes of relentless pain? Cigarette smoking, sugar, soda, citrus, white potatoes, and peanut butter. There may be others. What you put in your mouth becomes you. These items may be pain initiators, and cigarettes always slow the healing process.

Natural Prescription for Health: Stop and think before you eat: Does this food promote or subtract from my health bottom line?

Personal Thoughts/Goals:

_____

_____

_____

_____

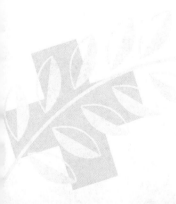

Day 280

Medical Reports

Men who walked for at least two hours a week had a twenty-five percent *lower risk* of getting an *enlarged prostate,* a benign condition that causes older men to urinate frequently.[48]

Waists matter more than hips or thighs, at least to your heart. Women under sixty with a thirty- to thirty-two-inch waist had *twice the risk of heart disease* as women whose waists measured less than twenty-eight inches. Women with at least a thirty-eight-inch waist had more than four times the risk.[49]

PC-SPES, a combination of herbs used by men with prostate cancer, has potent estrogen-like activity. Like estrogen, it *can lower levels of testosterone and PSA* (prostate specific antigen), but can also cause side effects (like breast tenderness and loss of libido).[50]

Mothers of children who were diagnosed with *brain tumors* were less likely to have taken *prenatal multivitamins* than mothers whose children did not develop brain tumors. However, it's possible that women who take vitamins also do something else that lowers their children's risk of brain tumors, like eating the right food and exercise. They may be more aware of the fact that what they eat affects their unborn child.[51]

> When I first came to see Dr. DeMaria, I had stomach pains and constipation and took antacids regularly. I had deterioration of the neck and couldn't move, just pain. It was difficult, but following Dr. Bob's advice I have stopped smoking and eliminated sugar from my diet, and I no longer drink alcohol. I still have a bit of constipation, but my neck is ninety-five percent better and so am I! —Katie O'Connor

Personal Thoughts/Goals:

_____

_____

_____

_____

Day 281

Overcoming Gravity

And let the beauty of the Lord our God be upon us, and establish the work of our hands for us… (Psalm 90:17).

Jesus said in John 16:33 that in the world you will have *tribulation,* which is translated into English from the Greek word *thlipsis. Thlipsis* is pressure—as in the pressure applied in an olive press. Jesus went on to say, *"Be of good cheer, I have overcome* [thlipsis].*"* You can experience *thlipsis* on your nervous system because of gravity pressing bones on sensitive nerves with poor posture, injuries, and the stresses of everyday living.

I call this *thlipsis* pressure on nerves *subluxation.* It is corrected and maintained by gentle laying on of the hands, adjusting the misalignment. In Mark 6:2 the people were astonished, saying, *"…And what wisdom is this which is given to Him, that such mighty works are performed by His hands!"* Are you under intense pressure? Tired of medication that covers and masks symptoms? It is time—you need to seek a godly, Jesus-filled, natural, spinal adjusting specialist!

We consult with worldwide clients via the Internet and telephone consultations. Go to www.druglessdoctor.com for details. Go to YouTube.com/druglessdoctor for timely videos. Follow us on Facebook at the DruglessDoctor or Twitter @druglessdoctor.

Natural Prescription for Health: Poor health? Poor posture? Seek a God-fearing, skilled spinal adjuster.

Personal Thoughts/Goals:

_____

_____

_____

_____

Day 282

The Riddle of Right Knee Pain

Therefore strengthen the hands which hang down, and the feeble knees
(Hebrews 12:12).

"But the natural man does not receive the things of the Spirit of God, for they are foolishness to Him; nor can He know them, because they are spiritually discerned" (1 Cor. 2:14). The human body is one interdependent contiguous tissue. I see a variety of conditions in my practice—knee pain can be baffling. Carrying more weight on one foot due to trunk alignment imbalance stresses the knees. Pain on the inside of the knee can be decay or cartilage and ligament tearing. General knee cap pain may be bursitis. Daily taking flax oil (one tablespoon per one hundred pounds of body weight), 150 milligrams B6, and organic apple cider vinegar relieves bursitis.

The real cause of outside right knee pain can only be gallbladder dysfunction. There is a Chinese acupuncture point located at the knee crease. It is not on the left knee. Does peanut butter, fries, fried chicken, or meat consumption correlate with knee pain? Eat a half apple daily. Use the castor oil pack on your liver once a week. I also suggest a bile salt supplement: one daily, then two, then three, then back to one.

Natural Prescription for Health: Flex the muscles in the front of your thighs for five seconds, three minutes daily to strengthen the knee.

Personal Thoughts/Goals:

_____

_____

_____

_____

Day 283

Pillar of Salt

But his [Lot's] *wife looked back behind him, and she became a pillar of salt*
(Genesis 19:26).

God created the physical body from the dust of the ground. We are made from dirt. Dirt has nutrients including minerals. Plants or vegetation take the inorganic material that humans are unable to process for optimal use and converts it to organic. I instruct my patients that minerals from plants and animals appear to be more easily absorbed and utilized in their natural complex state versus a synthetic, human-made pill. Assimilating nutrients needed for health are generally not available in synthetic sources.

I observe people moving when I am out and about shopping. Recently I noticed several individuals who appeared as pillars of salt. Their spines did not want to move freely. This is a result of many factors including subluxated or misaligned vertebrae that have been stuck for years. The body, through mechanism of repair, sends additional material to assist the healing process. Over time, the spine moves as one lump of petrified wood.

Natural Prescription for Health: Regular spinal assessment and correction is necessary for motion just like the car alignment of your vehicle frame. Tires and spines last longer when properly aligned.

Personal Thoughts/Goals:

_____

_____

_____

_____

Day 284

Be All You Can Be

Your garments did not wear out on you, nor did your foot swell these forty years
(Deuteronomy 8:4).

Jesus came to give us life to the fullest, to live in abundance. We are the builders of God's Kingdom on the earth. Chronic, repetitive stress can be annoying and, in fact, disabling. It is challenging to give one hundred percent if you don't feel one hundred percent. I commonly see areas of pain in the body caused by an injury or trauma which may seem insignificant but create relentless pain. Pain in the chest area after a twisting activity, like raking, can be caused by a rib that is out of alignment. Seek a spinal adjuster to correct the alignment. Wear shoes with arch support. Poor footwear can create ankle, knee, hip, and back pain. Flexibility is helpful; stretch daily; touch your toes and perform side bends.

I encourage eating alfalfa sprouts and tablets as a source of sodium. You need sodium to have pliable muscles and tissues. Pain can be caused by potentially many reasons. Focus on items you eat that create pain. A recent patient ate caramel popcorn that irritated his neck.

Natural Prescription for Health: Add quality oil on your salads including flax, rice, olive, and coconut oils; green veggies promote pain relief.

Personal Thoughts/Goals:

_____

_____

_____

_____

Day 285

Stay Connected to the Source

Abide in Me and I in you. As the branch cannot bear fruit by itself, unless it abides in the vine, neither can you, unless you abide in Me (John 15:4).

We all need to be connected to the vine—Jesus. Without Jesus, we can do nothing. Use your observation senses; seek and find a branch with barnacles connected to the trunk. Do you know why the barnacles are growing on the branch? It has become cellularly disconnected. A small trauma or injury could have weakened the branch, and microorganisms may have attacked the weakened tissue and the branch died. So why do we want to attach ourselves to a dead branch?

Mother nature uses barnacles, insects, and live organisms to dissolve the branch to be recycled. You too can become disconnected from the source by trauma or injury. When a vertebra moves and compresses a nerve, whatever tissue the nerve innervated will stop working at one hundred percent. Pharmaceuticals are designed to treat the symptoms caused by the power being shut off. Have you been plagued with poor health, including but not limited to chronic sinusitis, heart palpitations, bronchitis, asthma, digestive distress, constipation, diarrhea, menstrual pain, headaches, chronic neck pain, and earaches? Have you tried a variety of remedies and there is little to no improvement in your condition? Then it is time to be checked for subluxation by a skilled natural spinal specialist.

Natural Prescription for Health: Do you have chronic health issues? Is your postural aligned? If not, seek spinal corrective care.

Personal Thoughts/Goals:

_____

_____

_____

_____

Day 286

Feet Were Made to Walk

Ponder the path of your feet, and let all your ways be established (Proverbs 4:26).

Feet must be really important if Jesus took the time to wash the feet of His disciples. I know it was a symbolic gesture of serving, but there are other body parts. Did you ever stub your little toe? It hurts like crazy, and it alters your walking pace and pattern.

Do you know—this may sound farfetched—that you can get indigestion because of a misaligned foot bone. Yes. I have manually corrected a subluxated foot bone called the talus. The foot bone is connected to the ankle bone, which is connected to the knee, hip, and pelvis. The lumbar spine affects the muscles associated with hiatal hernia. Correcting the foot position impacts the entire body.

A common foot issue is tarsal tunnel (pain on the inside of your ankle) which responds to vitamin B6, 150 milligrams daily, and one tablespoon of flax per one hundred pounds of body weight. Toe fungus is a sign of a deep yeast infestation that can be helped with Agrisept, a citric seed extract.

Natural Prescription for Health: Heel pain with or without findings of a spur generally responds to a no-citrus diet and weight reduction. Add an ounce of organic apple cider vinegar to your salad dressing daily for one month.

Personal Thoughts/Goals:

_____

_____

_____

_____

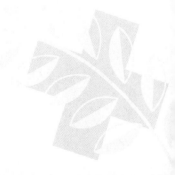

Day 287

TV Trouble

Watching TV can be hazardous to your health. In a recent study of more than fifty thousand women, every two hours per day of TV watching increased the risk of obesity by twenty-three percent and the risk of diabetes by fourteen percent. Sitting while at work was linked to much smaller increases in risk.

In contrast, every hour per day of brisk walking was linked to a twenty-four percent drop in the risk of obesity and a thirty-four percent drop in the risk of diabetes. An estimated thirty percent of new cases of obesity and forty-three percent of new cases of diabetes could be prevented if women would spend less than ten hours a week watching TV and at least thirty minutes a day walking briskly, say the authors of the study.[52]

Natural Prescription for Health: Get off the couch and go for a walk.

My family first came to see Dr. DeMaria due to frequent illnesses with the kids requiring trips to the doctor, prescription antibiotics, and ibuprofen. My daughter also had frequent migraine headaches. Dr. Bob recommended various lifestyle changes, all of which were difficult for the children; they were very resistant to change. As a family, we have made various diet changes. We now use natural sugar and organic foods. We no longer consume processed foods, "pop," or fast food. We also use all-natural remedies for illnesses. These changes have made the children happier and healthier, whether they will admit it or not. —Cynthia Bublenic

Personal Thoughts/Goals:

_____

_____

_____

_____

Day 288

Subluxation

These things I have spoken to you, that in Me you may have peace. In the world you will have tribulation [thlipsis]; *but be of good cheer, I have overcome the world* (John 16:33).

When God created people, He breathed life into us so we are self-healing beings. Our brains are so intricately created with so many options that we will never even capitalize on its full capacity. A continuation of the brain is the spinal cord, which is encased in a moveable conduit called the spinal column. Gravity continuously and relentlessly compresses the twenty-four moveable vertebrae making the column. Humans are bipeds (standing on two legs), which causes tremendous pressure on fulcrum points—the neck, mid and low back.

Motion is essential for life. Injury to the spine results in trauma, which is *thlipsis* or pressure. Neurothlipsis, or a vertebral subluxation, is when a bone is compressing or choking nerves, reducing the flow of life or energy from the brain to tissue cells. Correcting subluxation and strengthening and improving *posture* will result in an improved level of optimal health. Seek a natural spinal adjuster.

Natural Prescription for Health: Look at your full posture today. Close your eyes, tilt your head, back and forth. Open them. Look in the mirror. Now does you head shift? Is your neck centered and shoulders level? Have someone take a side posture view with a digital camera; your ear should be perpendicular to your shoulder—use your drawing mode and draw a line from the shoulder up and place a dot in your ear. Every inch your ear is anterior to the line from the shoulder adds ten pounds of extra head weight to the base of your neck.

Personal Thoughts/Goals:

_____

_____

_____

_____

Day 289

What's in Front of Your Eyes?

*And I, Daniel, alone saw the vision, for the men who were
with me did not see the vision…* (Daniel 10:7).

Elijah saw in the spirit what his servant could not see until he prayed for his eyes to be opened. Daniel, Jacob, and Paul saw a vision. My prayer is for you to have your eyes opened for your health's sake. The power that made the body—our Heavenly Father—breathed life into us to heal the body.

I seek and correct spinal misplacements in my patients. When a vertebra is out of its relationship with the one above or below, it compresses the nerves that leave the spinal canal. I call that a subluxation. Your body works by information being sent from the brain cell to the tissue cell. If you have a long-term health issue that has not resolved on its own or with medication, it is highly probable that the power switch or vertebra has moved, interrupting the messages from the main body computer or brain. We see miracles daily involving long-term conditions that resolve over time with natural spinal corrective care.

Natural Prescription for Health: Look at your posture. If you are not aligned and centered, seek a spinal subluxation specialist.

Personal Thoughts/Goals:

_____

_____

_____

_____

Day 290

Joints

And not holding fast to the Head, from whom all the body…[is] nourished and knit together by joints and ligaments… (Colossians 2:19).

The Word of God is living and powerful, sharper than a two-edged sword, capable of separating joints and marrow. Joints have been designed to be strong and carry our weight, and they are used for motion. Motion is life. Pain, severe intense joint pain, cripples a significant segment of society.

Sulfur and other minerals and elements are used by the body for joint strength. Sulfur helps make collagen a critical factor for joint, skin, muscle, and ligament strength. Excellent sources of sulfur include *eggs, onion, garlic, radishes,* and *cabbage.* A heavy phlegm in the throat is a body signal of a sulfur deficiency. Also a deepening of your voice is a sign of low sulfur. Sulfur is actually stored in the tonsils. Smokers generally have low sulfur, which is a reason their skin is always so drawn or worn. Sulfur makes skin elastic. I also see joint pain with milk consumption.

Natural Prescription for Health: Water is an excellent lubricant and natural way to relieve pain. Add sulfur foods and water and minimize dairy.

Personal Thoughts/Goals:

_____

_____

_____

_____

Day 291

Life Without Medication

Let our Master now command your servants, who are before you, to seek out a man who is a skillful player on the harp. And it shall be that he will play it with his hand when the distressing spirit from God is upon you and you shall be well (1 Samuel 16:16).

Body signals with pain can be relieved without medication, but an action step is required. Pain can be caused by a distressing spirit from the Lord. Saul was disobedient to the command of the Lord; therefore, obedience is more important than sacrifice. *"The Spirit of the Lord departed from Saul, and a distressing spirit from the Lord troubled him"* (1 Sam. 16:14).

Is a distressing spirit holding you hostage? Seek the Lord for healing.

Is anyone among you suffering? Let him pray. Is anyone cheerful? Let him sing psalms. Is anyone among you sick? Let him call for the elders of the church and let them pray over him, anointing him with oil in the name of the Lord. And the prayer of faith will save the sick, and the Lord will raise him up. And if he committed sins, he will be forgiven (James 5:13-15).

Divine healing may be exactly what the doctor ordered. I pray you are receiving the healing you are seeking.

Natural Prescription for Health: Seek counsel from a sincere spiritual leader in your church community.

Personal Thoughts/Goals:

_____

_____

_____

_____

Day 292

Personal Evolution

*For everyone who partakes only of milk is unskilled in the word of righteousness,
for he is a babe. But solid food belongs to those who are of full age, that is, those who
by **reason of use** have their senses exercised to discern both good and evil*
(Hebrews 5:13-14, emphasis added).

Achieving new levels of health takes courage in a culture where billions of prescriptions are consumed. Peak performance requires energy and the capacity to change or else you will continue in the same downward spiral of poor health.

Are you on antidepressants? Focus on increasing flax oil, one tablespoon per one hundred pounds body weight. Add more protein, along with 150 milligrams of B6 a day for three months. Do you suffer with constipation? Increase your water consumption and raw vegetables. If you constantly deal with chronic sinus problems, eliminate dairy and peanut butter. Shoulder pain can be corrected by eliminating citrus. Do you have morning headaches? Cease eating sweet fruit or sweet snacks before bed. Chocolate cravings? Eat mixed green salads daily. To curb your desire for dairy, try focusing on olive and flax oil for fat along with sesame seeds for calcium and protein. Are you struggling to lose weight? Drink more water and minimize your sweets. Sweets increase insulin. You will have challenges losing weight with elevated insulin. Leg cramps while sleeping can be eliminated by adding sesame seeds and almonds to your diet.

Natural Prescription for Health: Discern labels while shopping. Avoid trans fat, high fructose corn syrup, and sugar.

Personal Thoughts/Goals:

_____

_____

_____

_____

Day 293

Tennis Elbow

He has shown strength with His arm... (Luke 1:51).

God showed strength in His arm by protecting His people Israel. The arm of the Lord protects us today from satan. Arms can be used for offensive and defensive purposes.

Arm pain, especially elbow pain, prevents even the basic of human functions. Elbow pain on the outside aspect is seen in motions of twisting the arm and hand, as in hitting a tennis ball. The structures involved are normally tendons and its coverings. The condition is tenosynovitis. Applying pressure on the traumatized site can send you through the roof with pain. We use a narrow elastic sleeve two inches below the elbow crease to change the fulcrum point. This allows healing to occur at the elbow.

Yes, take a break from tennis. For chronic pain, supplement your diet with a anchovy/sardine-based marine oil for three weeks, taking two teaspoons a day for three weeks; then take only flax oil with a whole food B6 (150 milligrams daily), and apple cider vinegar, one tablespoon a day. The elbow joint may require mobilization by a skilled practitioner experienced in natural joint manipulation.

Natural Prescription for Health: Minimize citrus consumption if you experience elbow pain.

Personal Thoughts/Goals:

_____

_____

_____

_____

Day 294

Liposuction: No Heart Saver

Liposuction can remove fat cells, but—unlike diet and exercise—may not cut your risk of heart disease and diabetes.

Researchers removed roughly twenty pounds of mostly abdominal fat from fifteen obese women (each had at least a forty-inch waist). But after ten to twelve weeks, there was no change in their insulin resistance, blood sugar, blood pressure, cholesterol, C-reactive protein, or other risk factors for heart disease.[53]

Natural Prescription for Health: If you're overweight, eat less and exercise more. Liposuction may shed pounds—but not risk. It doesn't make you take in fewer calories than you burn. Another possibility? Although it removes fat cells that are subcutaneous (just under the skin), liposuction doesn't shrink fat cells or remove the fat that's deeper in the abdomen, liver, and muscles.

> I had been suffering with a stressed Achilles tendon, plantars fuscia, bursitis, and sore left hip with numbness to my entire left leg. I also was very stressed and fatigued and had trouble sleeping. The information and care provided by Dr. DeMaria has improved my stress/fatigue. I now sleep better at night, and I'm back to running without the after pain. I am now more cautious of what I eat and how much sugar I consume. Thank you for making my life less stressful! I highly recommend your services to my family and friends.
> —Dianne Shrenkel

Personal Thoughts/Goals:

_____

_____

_____

_____

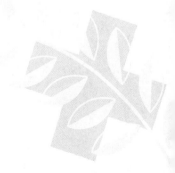

Restful, Peaceful Sleep

Your body repairs itself during restful, peaceful sleep. Plan your daily routine; manage your time in such a way that you are in bed before midnight. Avoid activities that are not productive. Procrastination steals sleep time. Have a sleep schedule that is consistent with your meal planning, exercise, and quiet time.

Day 295

Deep Sleep

And the Lord caused a deep sleep to fall on Adam, and he slept (Genesis 2:21).

The best sleep is a deep, God sleep. Adam and Saul both were in a deep sleep, Adam for a rib to be removed to create woman and Saul for David's safety. Sleep is when your body has the opportunity to do all the repairs.

People today with the rush of life, stress, and anxiety generally do not get the sleep they need. Many work two jobs to make ends meet. Single parents with children are especially challenged. I encourage patients to exercise during the day, if possible. Exercise promotes movement and cleansing of fluids and toxins. Endorphins released during exercise create an atmosphere of calmness. Calcium citrate and lactate help people fall asleep and prevent leg cramps at night. Turkey and tuna have tryptophan, which is a sleep precursor. Caffeine creates a problem when your liver is not capable of clearing its stimulating effects.

Natural Prescription for Health: Eat sesame seeds, calcium lactate, or citrate with a turkey or tuna dinner as sources of calcium and tryptophan to promote initial sleep drowsiness.

Personal Thoughts/Goals:

_____

_____

_____

_____

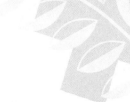

Day 296

Laughter—God's Heart Medicine

…We were like those who dream. Then our mouth was filled with laughter, and our tongue with singing (Psalm 126:1-2)

The heart of the physical person in a busy life receives enormous stress from diet and lifestyle choices. Do you take time to laugh? Laughter is God's medicine for the heart. Laughter relaxes blood vessels boosting blood flow. Life is in the blood. It carries essential nutrients and oxygen to tissue cells. Mental stress causes blood vessels to constrict or get smaller, reducing blood flow. When you laugh, reactions in the body are prompted by a release of nitric oxide, which relaxes blood vessels much like endorphins released during exercise. When you laugh, you also have less wear on your joints.

A good belly laugh a day would be a step toward heart health. Rent or purchase some of your favorite programs on DVD—watching something wholesome and entertaining is sure safer than taking medications.

Natural Prescription for Health: Look at old family and friend pictures on your desk top, tablet, or phone. Have some fun and "face time" or "video chat" with friends and family. Share the experience!

Personal Thoughts/Goals:

_____

_____

_____

_____

Day 297

Tissue Repairs Occur During Sleep

...Both the chariot and horse were cast into a dead sleep (Psalm 76:6).

Restful, peaceful sleep without interruption of natural body function is essential to promote organ and tissue revitalization. Poor calcium utilization and resulting deficiencies prevent the initial calmness to achieve initial sleep.

Leg cramping while lying down at night is a common body signal suggesting a need for calcium. Sesame seeds, almonds, and mixed greens added to your diet would be a good start as they are easily assimilated by the body. If you are currently taking an over-the-counter calcium supplement and have night leg cramps, try another product with calcium citrate or lactate. Avoid digestive aid calcium products that contain calcium carbonate; they are more difficult to absorb.

Stress and sunshine deplete the body reserves of calcium.

Natural Prescription for Health: The hours in bed *before* midnight promote healing and restoration. Sleep six to eight hours each night.

Personal Thoughts/Goals:

_____

_____

_____

_____

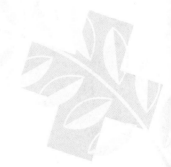

Day 298

Depression Freedom

Anxiety in the heart of man causes depression, but a good word makes it glad
(Proverbs 12:25).

Feeding on the Word of God fills a void; without the Word, people are empty.

A leading cause of depression is a lack of quality nutrients in the diet. An organic source of Omega 3 flax oil (one tablespoon per day per one hundred pounds body weight) promotes the formation of DHA needed for brain health. Whole food B vitamins and minerals create an environment for emotional stability.

Eliminate sugar from your life. Sugar robs the body of substances needed to complete the formation of fat for brain activity. Human-made trans fat or partially and hydrogenated fats sabotage every cell reaction and can lead to emotional imbalance, including ADHD. Exercise promotes "feel good" endorphin production in the body, which reduces anxiety.

Read God's Word daily. Filling your heart with the Word leaves no room for depression.

Natural Prescription for Health: Depressed? For emotional stability take either two teaspoons of an anchovy/sardine-sourced marine oil or one tablespoon of flax oil per one hundred pounds of body weight. Essential Fatty Acid or EFA blood spot test is a wise test to allowing you to create the proper fat/oil supplementation protocol.

Personal Thoughts/Goals:

_____

_____

_____

_____

Day 299

Sweet Sleep

After this I awoke and looked around, and my sleep was so sweet to me
(Jeremiah 31:26).

Rest and/or peace elude many people today. Prescription medication may be a part of the cause. Prior asthma patients often tell me that they did not always sleep through the night while on their medication. It was only after eliminating the medication and changing their diets that they slept peacefully.

Elevated tissue copper levels may keep your brain racing even if your body is exhausted. Increasing calcium-rich food sources (like sesame seeds, almonds, and mixed greens) helps. Low calcium may prevent drowsiness. Consuming turkey and tuna increases natural sources of tryptophan, a necessary ingredient for sleep. Minimize caffeinated products, including the obvious coffee and tea, but also chocolate. You need optimal liver function to process caffeine. Over-the-counter pain remedies may also be a part of your dilemma.

Exercise helps calm the body. Also, forgive and settle any emotional issues.

Natural Prescription for Health: Add organic turkey to your menus.

Personal Thoughts/Goals:

_____

_____

_____

_____

Day 300

The Lamp of Your Body

The lamp of the body is the eye. If, therefore, your eye is good,
your whole body will be full of light (Matthew 6:22).

Light penetrates to the back of the eye. You actually see with your brain through the two "video cams," or your eyes. Jesus healed the blind. You can be physically and spiritually blind since the natural person does not receive the things of the Spirit of God (see 1 Cor. 2:14). Your ability to receive sunlight is affected by your mineral level consumption. I have had patients who lack the mineral potassium who appear to have a slower pupil response. The dark spot in the colored part of the eye is affected by what you eat and what causes you stress.

Does bright light bother your eyes? Eat less sugar and eat more cucumbers. Trouble driving at night? Eat more carrots. Are your eyes dry? Try iodine first for three months and potassium if that does not help. Are cataracts blurring your vision? Have your calcium and phosphorus level checked by your healthcare provider. The ratio should be ten parts calcium to four parts phosphorous. An imbalance with excessive calcium may result in a cloudy lens. We encourage eating grains and protein to lower the calcium. Eat whole foods.

Natural Prescription for Health: Soda consumption can imbalance your phosphorous level. The nightshades including tomatoes, potatoes, green pepper, and eggplant can interrupt normal calcium and phosphorous balance.

Personal Thoughts/Goals:

_____

_____

_____

_____

Day 301

Sleep and Aging

"For many years, we've known that sleep in older people is very different from sleep in younger people," says Julie Carrier of the Sleep Center at the Sacre-Coeur Hospital in Montreal. "Starting at 30 years of age, complaints about sleep increase, and they continue into a person's 80s."

There's a reason for that. "Older people have almost no slow-wave sleep," she says. "That's the deepest stage, when people sleep very, very soundly. What's more, as you age you wake up more often and have more trouble getting back to sleep."

Older people also have problems adapting to changes in sleep time, says Carrier. "They have a lot more complaints about the effects of shift work or jet lag. We believe that the sleep-wake cycle becomes more fragile, more vulnerable to disruptions."

Then there's menopause. "Hot flashes aside, complaints about sleep are one of the biggest problems reported by menopausal women," says Carrier. "Yet there are very few objective studies that try to understand why women have so many problems falling and staying asleep during menopause."

What can older people do to improve their sleep? "Try to take care of your sleep-wake cycle," says Carrier. "Go to bed and get up at the same time each day."[54]

Natural Prescription for Health: Hot flashes respond to a source of organic iodine. Men and women would do well to increase protein during the day to assist the body in having enough sleep-inducing tryptophan.

> I believe that Dr. DeMaria saved my life! Previously I had sinus issues and felt crazy. I wasn't able to work and was sleepy all day. I took lots of Sudafed, Tylenol, Allegra, and Singular. Dr. Bob encouraged me to quit smoking after twenty-seven years. I have no more sinus issues, and I feel like a new woman with lots more energy. It was difficult to quit smoking, but thanks to Dr. Bob, I did quit and feel wonderful! Dr. Bob has also helped my children. —Tracy Lewis

Personal Thoughts/Goals:

_____

_____

_____

_____

Day 302

Rest in the Lord

Rest in the Lord, and wait patiently for Him (Psalm 37:7).

God, yes God, rested on the seventh day. He created the entire universe; then He rested. (See Genesis 2:2.) Wow! If God rested, that is definitely a mandate for us to rest.

A couple of tips: Stress and anxiety interrupt a normal pattern of sleep. If you have difficulty achieving sleep, try shutting off the television and stop reading the news. Play soothing instrumental praise and worship music to calm the spirit. Let your brain have a break from noise as it settles down for the evening. Do you wake up two hours after you fall asleep? Take a whole food B vitamin before you lay your head down. I encourage flat or low pillows so your head is not raised but horizontal to the bed. Cover the alarm, VCR, and TV lights in your room. They disrupt deep sleep. Minimize caffeine before bed.

Do you or your spouse snore? Put a wedge of lemon in hot water and sip on it. Then eat the lemon. Place your troubles with the Lord.

Natural Prescription for Health: Cover all the lights in your bedroom while sleeping—alarm clock, fire/carbon monoxide alarms, night lights, your TV, audio and video equipment. Glowing light from the simplest source can disrupt normal sleep patterns. Waking up hungry is a positive body signal that your body is creating growth hormone—which suggests healing is occurring.

Personal Thoughts/Goals:

_____

_____

_____

_____

Day 303

Pray for Perception

*Be aware of false prophets who come in sheep's clothing,
but inwardly they are ravenous wolves* (Matthew 7:15).

I read *The Wall Street Journal* regularly. It has given me an interesting perception on health issues. Jesus was constantly raising the apostles' awareness of the Pharisees and Sadducees. They appeared to be lovers of God, but in fact, they were self-lovers. Economics has a lot to do with health. The industry, affected by decisions on health research, will complain and minimize reports that negatively affect them. Heart disease, cancer, Alzheimer's, digestive distress, and depression are affected by the politics of health. You are in the middle unless you are perceptive. WWJD? He would, as in many cases throughout His ministry, be countercultural. The Word says to eat food from plants that yield seed, no genetically-modified food. Therefore, eat certified organic food. Avoid human-made foods, including human-made substitutes for sugar and fat. Eat the real thing.

Natural Prescription for Health: God-made maple syrup and honey are the best choices for sweeteners. Olive and flax oil are your best fats of choice.

Personal Thoughts/Goals:

_____

_____

_____

_____

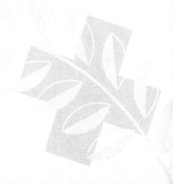

Day 304

Solid Foundation

Therefore, whoever hears these sayings of Mine, and does them, I will liken him to a wise man who built his house on the rock (Matthew 7:24).

I love the way the Lord spoke to the people. He did not mince words. Life principles, spiritual and physical, are logical and are best followed. Would you build a house on sand? Certainly not—unless you were from another planet! The Word of God, Jesus, is your spiritual foundation, the Cornerstone.

Your body's foundation is the bone framework. Soda, smoking, and aspirin weaken bones. Yes, aspirin slows bone healing. The phosphoric acid in soda, which creates bubbles, leaches calcium. Smoking depletes minerals and precious vitamin C. Excellent bone builders include calcium and protein. My experience suggests that calcium sourced from plants and seeds does not alter the acid state in the body and need to be neutralized. Sesame seeds and almonds are the first choice. Chicken, fish, turkey, and beans make great sources of protein. Walking, light fitness training, and Pilates create bone stress for calcium to go to the bone matrix.

Natural Prescription for Health: Add calcium from plant sources daily.

Personal Thoughts/Goals:

_____

_____

_____

_____

Day 305

Time Well Spent

And the Lord said to [Ananias], *"Arise and go to the street called Straight, and inquire at the house of Judas for one called Saul of Tarsas, for behold, he is praying"* (Acts 9:11).

It's been said that you will be the exact same person in five years, except for two events that occur in your life—the people you meet and the books you read. Twenty-four hours speed along into weeks, weeks into months, and months into years. The twelve apostles met Jesus. They were different. The Pharisees were confounded by the depth of knowledge Jesus had without formal education.

I challenge you to start reading at least one new book every month. Read books that promote spiritual or physical life. Avoid books that only entertain or amuse you. Pray for new people to come into your fellowship circle. Take time to write the exact attributes in a person you want to associate with. Create time in your schedule to expand your inner circle to a larger circle. The Lord has new friends for you. Paul (Saul) was visited by Ananias, who changed his life.

Natural Prescription for Health: Read one new book this month. Cultivate one new solid relationship with someone this year.

Personal Thoughts/Goals:

_____

_____

_____

_____

Day 306

The Cheerful Giver

So let each one give as he purposes in his heart, not grudgingly or of necessity; for God loves a cheerful giver (2 Corinthians 9:7).

God so loved the world that He gave His only begotten son, so we may have eternal life. (See John 3:16.) Give and it shall be given to you. To get a friend, be a friend. Take the focus of your life off of you.

Now hear me on this. Position your life to give, help, and teach. No doubt you've heard the saying: Give a man a fish; feed a man for a day. Teach a man to fish; feed him for a lifetime. It's true that life skills are necessary for a happy, successful life. There are times in people's lives when, because of their poor choices, you may need to give them support to prevent a crisis. On the other hand, continued giving and support may not always be wise—a little tough love and discipline may be the answer. The prodigal son had to come to his senses in his own time. Confrontation of issues may be in order.

Giving is God's economy. Help those in need. Be a blessing to someone anonymously now, and you will be rewarded in Heaven later.

Natural Prescription for Health: Find someone or an organization and give of your resources.

Personal Thoughts/Goals:

_____

_____

_____

_____

Day 307

Stool Secrets

*Are you thus without understanding also? Do you not perceive that whatever enters a man from the outside cannot defile him, because it does not enter his heart, but his stomach, and is **eliminated**, thus purifying all foods?* (Mark 7:18-19, emphasis added).

Jesus spoke of what came from the heart. The thoughts and emotions of the hearts of people defile them.

Stools or bowel movements are a signature of your health. My colon therapist tells her clients that regular daily bowel elimination is to occur after meals. Stools that sink indicate a need for more oil in the diet. Foul-smelling stools occur with poor digestion and slow removal.

Fiber increases the passage of the food. You don't get adequate fiber from white bread, doughnuts, fries, and pastries. Regular consistent fiber food, especially apples, are good for the colon. Fiber gently scrapes the colon walls. Psyllium tends to absorb too much water, dehydrating the colon. Flax fiber and powder is a better choice. Diarrhea may be a sign of lactose issues or even toxicity.

Natural Prescription for Health: Eat mixed greens to increase magnesium, causing better transit time. Avoid dependence on laxatives.

Personal Thoughts/Goals:

_____

_____

_____

_____

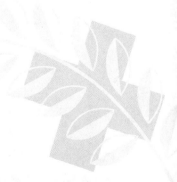

Day 308

Baths and Sleep

A hot bath before bedtime raises the body's temperature, and the subsequent cooling may trigger sleep. In the first study of baths for the treatment of insomnia, nine women insomniacs in their sixties and seventies took hot baths an hour and a half before bedtime.

"The women reported deeper sleep, less restlessness during the night, and more rested in the morning after a hot bath than after a bath at body temperature, which they perceived as 'cool,'" reports Cynthia Dorsey of the Sleep Disorders Center and Sleep Research Program at McLean Hospital in Belmont, Massachusetts. Measurements of brain activity confirmed that the women awakened less during the night.[55]

Natural Prescription for Health: A hot bath with mineral salts will help calm the tissues and is an excellent source of minerals. Avoid toxic-sourced bubble bath compounds.

> I had various health complaints before making Dr. DeMaria's recommended lifestyle changes. I suffered with depression, shoulder pain, and leg pain. I could write a book about what Dr. Bob has taught me. We are responsible for our actions. Be aware of what you do, eat, and exercise. —Gerald F. Teggart

Personal Thoughts/Goals:

_____

_____

_____

_____

Day 309

Stay Strong

*And the Lord said, 'Simon, Simon! Indeed, Satan has asked for you that he may sift you as wheat. But I have **prayed** for you, that your faith should not fail; and when you have returned to Me, strengthen your brethren* (Luke 22:31-32, emphasis added).

Jesus very calmly said this to His protégé, Peter, and He prayed for his protection when satan *requested* to persecute him. Jesus was a prayer warrior for Peter in a time of need. Be a prayer warrior for one of your own today. Satan searches to and fro seeking someone to devour (see 1 Pet. 5:8).

Being strong physically is necessary to staying strong spiritually. It is much more of a challenge to do the Lord's work when you are physically exhausted. There are three, eight-hour "segment days" in one twenty-four-hour day. Use them to nourish and feed your spiritual and physical self. When your feet first hit the floor (after seven to eight hours of sleep) is "Day 1" of the first segment. This is a good time to "sharpen the saw" with exercise, reading God's Word, prayer, getting your day focused, and eating a nutritious breakfast. "Day 2" of the three segments is when you start work until your shift is over, regardless of your profession. Give 110 percent to your livelihood. "Day 3" of the three-in-one day begins when your work duties are completed until you go to bed. The hours in bed sleeping before midnight are significant.

Spend time with your family and friends. Minimize the time you are entertained by media. Initiating this lifestyle promotes spiritual and physical strength.

Natural Prescription for Health: "Early to bed, early to rise, makes a man healthy, wealthy, and wise." —Benjamin Franklin

Personal Thoughts/Goals:

_____

_____

_____

_____

Day 310

Seasoned With Salt

Let your speech always be with grace, seasoned with salt that you may know how you...answer each one (Colossians 4:6).

Paul was encouraging the Colossians to use wisdom and wholesome speech in conversation with non-Christians. I thoroughly enjoy how Paul uses the metaphor of salt.

Salt enhances the taste of food by drawing out the "au jus" from entrees. I encourage using natural Celtic Sea Salt; it has not been colored or chlorinated. Chlorine is often used by commercial brands to whiten their salt product. Aluminum, a known toxin when in abundance on neuron structures, and dextrose, a sugar, have been used as anticaking factors.

I am aware that sodium chloride, or standard table salt, has been used as a source of iodine, but I question the source of the commercial potassium iodine. Does it really assist the thyroid function? Why do we have so many low thyroid patients? Use Celtic Sea Salt on your food. Only five percent of blood pressure cases have been associated with salt.

Natural Prescription for Health: Homegrown herbs on your favorite dishes enhance the essence of the flavor.

Personal Thoughts/Goals:

_____

_____

_____

_____

Day 311

Shine as Lights in the World

Do all things without complaining and disputing, that you may become blameless and harmless children of God without fault in the midst of a crooked and perverse generation, among whom you shine as lights of the world (Philippians 2:14-15).

Whatever you do with these new patterns, please do not whine or complain. Learn to be an example. Make positive comments.

When I gave my life to the Lord, I continued to drink alcohol. I was released from alcohol four years later. Not only was alcohol no longer a part of my life, I also stopped eating sugar.

I see very unhealthy people almost every day. I attempt to avoid patterns that critically sick people practice. I discipline myself without focusing on the individuals with whom I am in contact with at events. When asked, I explain how sugar disrupts the immune system. You see, people get infections and lower resistance using sugar. Headaches, sinus problems, and bronchitis diminish when sugar is eliminated. Be a light to the world; share your knowledge in love.

Natural Prescription for Health: Do not make a big scene when you make a choice to make lifestyle modifications.

Personal Thoughts/Goals:

_____

_____

_____

_____

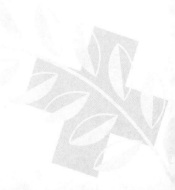

Day 312

Arise and Shine

Arise and shine; for your light has come! And the glory of the Lord is risen upon you
(Isaiah 60:1).

To quote Benjamin Franklin, "Early to bed, early to rise, makes a man healthy, wealthy, and wise." The hours you sleep before midnight are critical for optimal health. The adrenal gland, which is located on top of your kidneys, makes cortisone. When you go to bed late, your adrenal glands have to work harder. The adrenals will wear out over time. You may have pain and belly fat due to always having to get your "second wind."

Focus on being in bed by ten. Exercise during the day will help you be in a state to fall asleep. Turkey is an excellent source of trytophan needed to make a hormone for sleep. Minimize caffeine after dinner. Caffeine is found in chocolate, sodas, and some painkillers. Some teas even have more caffeine than coffee. Trouble falling asleep will improve by eating calcium-rich sesame seeds. You will get the best deep sleep when all light sources are eliminated.

I generally wake early, pray with my wife, read my Bible, and then exercise.

Natural Prescription for Health: Plan to be in bed sleeping by 10:00 p.m. and awake by 6:00 a.m. Use morning time to "sharpen your saw."

Personal Thoughts/Goals:

_____

_____

_____

_____

Day 313

Watch What You Touch

When the army goes out against your enemies, keep yourself from every wicked thing. …
But it shall be, when evening comes, that he shall wash with water…
(Deuteronomy 23:9,11).

In the Word of God, the nation of Israel was schooled and disciplined in their state of cleanliness. The guidelines that God gave Israel are intended to protect us, not to condemn us. The intertwining of the religious rules with rituals created a hierarchy of hatred and yokes difficult to break. Today, we live in an environment where we are only one, two, or three people away from the entire world. I have a friend in London, who was in Kenya, and he had friends from India.

I do not want you to become paranoid—just perceptive. Here are a few guidelines: Wash your hands, and watch what you put in your mouth. Only eat cooked food, not burnt, with no undercooked "au jus" or flesh present. Do not let children play in uncovered sandboxes. Be mindful of outside cats that eat mice. Do not eat sushi. If you have pain in your body after eating sushi, you need to be tested for parasites. Do not allow your children to play in toy lands that feature hundreds of plastic balls—fecal material and other parasite-transmitting debris may be present. Kids returning from petting zoos should have their clothes and hands washed properly.

Natural Prescription for Health: Do not consume any food item that has a decayed odor. No exceptions!

Personal Thoughts/Goals:

_____

_____

_____

_____

Day 314

Sickness Not Unto Death

This sickness is not unto death, but for the glory of God,
that the Son of God may be glorified through it (John 11:4).

The people at the time of Lazarus' apparent death and restoration surely were taken aback by the miracle Jesus performed. Various levels of sicknesses are rampant in our society today. I read an article about how minute toxins create disease. You would do best to focus on avoiding processed food. It is important to eat your liver-cleaning beets daily.

An interesting condition, not necessarily classified as a sickness, is insomnia. I also read how the aging population has challenges sleeping. Many resort to sleeping pills. To get a good night's sleep, I suggest exercise during the day and eating sesame seeds and almonds for a source of calcium.

Another issue I see regularly is annoying, itchy skin. A sickness? No—a sign of poor calcium tissue movement. Add flax oil to your meals. If you have difficulty swallowing, which is also quite common, eat potassium-rich cucumbers.

Natural Prescription for Health: Common health conditions nearly always respond to lifestyle modification

Personal Thoughts/Goals:

_____

_____

_____

_____

Day 315

Eat to Sleep

Most of us are probably convinced that what we eat and when we eat affects how well we sleep. Yet there's remarkably little research on the subject.

Do some foods make us drowsier than others? Does a nighttime snack help or hurt the odds of getting a good night's sleep? All we have are a few clues from short-term studies on a small number of people who had no sleep problems.

Young men fell asleep just as quickly within a few hours after a late-afternoon, high-fat meal as after a high-carbohydrate meal with the same number of calories. "There are lots of claims about this or that food," says Gary Zammit, Director of the Sleep Research Institute in New York. "But nothing stands out as being better than anything else."

A dinner of ordinary solid food put young men to sleep faster than a liquid dinner with the same number of calories.[56] Interesting, but it's not exactly proof that a handful of crackers will make you sleepier than a glass of milk.

Natural Prescription for Health: A source of wheat-free, no hydrogenated fat or trans fat crackers would be a good choice. Try sesame seed rice crackers. They provide an excellent source of calcium also.

> The back of my neck would tingle and hurt when I reached for something. My lower back especially would lock up, and I would be in severe pain. I would get bronchitis every year or so. I used ibuprofen on and off. Following Dr. DeMaria's advice, I am now eating less sugar. I take different supplements, and I try to eat better food sometimes. Cutting back on sugar has been difficult, but I am still trying to eat less sugar and still trying to buy less food with sugar in it. The information and care provided by Dr. Bob has helped me so that I can now walk without being in severe pain or having to take ibuprofen. My neck pain and tingling are gone. Because of the supplements and advice from Dr. Bob, I am much healthier and my immune system is stronger. —Elysse Saunders

Personal Thoughts/Goals:

_____

_____

_____

_____

"Saw" Sharpening

Daily self-improvement is essential for balanced health. The "saw" is you. Cutting blades are more efficient and effective when sharp. Read your Bible daily. Read an additional self-improvement book that is geared to your needs; listen to a teaching CD or watch a DVD a minimum of thirty minutes daily. While on an energizing walk, listen to praise music or commercial-free Christian music on a smart phone, MP3 player, or other audio equipment.

As mentioned previously, you will be the exact same person as you are today in five years except for the impact from the books you read and people you meet.

Sharpen your saw daily!

pH Chart

Eat eighty percent alkaline foods and twenty percent acid foods for perfect pH balance. Drink half an ounce of water per pound of body weight per day, not to exceed one hundred ounces, because of the need to flush toxins from the body. Not consuming enough water while on this program may result in a healing crisis.

References: *Acid & Alkaline* by Herman Aihara; *Alkalize Or Die* by Theodore A. Baroody, Ph.D., N.D. "Diets that are rich in animal foods and low in vegetable foods, typical of industrialized countries, lead to a dietary net acid load that has a negative effect on calcium balance" (*American Journal of Clinical Nutrition* 73 no. 1: 118).

Most Alkaline	Alkaline	Lowest Alkaline	Food Category	Lowest Acid	Acid	Most Acid
Stevia	Maple Syrup, Rice Syrup	Raw Honey, Raw Sugar	**Sweeteners**	Processed Honey, Molasses	White Sugar, Brown Sugar	NutraSweet, Equal, Sweet'n Low
Lemons, Watermelon, Limes, Grapefruit, Mangoes, Papayas	Dates/Figs, Melons, Grapes, Papaya, Kiwi, Berries, Apples, Pears, Raisins	Oranges, Bananas, Cherries, Pineapple, Peaches, Avocados	**Fruits**	Plums, Processed Fruit Juices	Sour Cherries, Rhubarb	Blueberries, Cranberries, Prunes
Asparagus, Onions, Vegetable Juices, Parsley, Raw Spinach, Broccoli, Garlic	Okra, Squash, Green Beans, Beets, Celery, Lettuce, Zucchini, Sweet Potato	Carrots, Tomatoes, Fresh Corn, Mushrooms, Cabbage, Peas, Potato Skins, Olives	**Beans, Vegetables, Legumes**	Spinach, Kidney Beans, String Beans	Potatoes, Pinto Beans, Navy Beans, Lima Beans	Soybean, Carob
	Almonds	Chestnuts	**Nuts/Seeds**	Pumpkin Seeds, Sunflower Seeds	Pecans, Cashews	Peanuts, Walnuts
Olive Oil	Flax Oil	Canola Oil	**Oils**	Corn Oil		
		Amaranth, Miller, Wild Rice, Quinoa	**Grains, Cereals**	Sprouted Wheat Bread, Spelt, Brown Rice	White Rice, Corn, Buckwheat, Oats, Rye	Wheat, White Flour, Pastries, Pasta
			Meats	Venison, Cold Water Fish	Turkey, Chicken, Lamb	Pork, Beef, Shellfish
	Breast Milk	Goat Milk, Goat Cheese, Whey	**Eggs, Dairy**	Eggs, Butter/ Yogurt, Buttermilk, Cottage Cheese	Soy Cheese, Raw Milk, Soy Milk	Cheese, Homogenized Milk, Ice Cream
Lemon, Water, Herb Teas	Green Tea	Ginger Tea	**Beverages**	Tea	Coffee	Beer, Soft Drinks

Day 316

Synthetic Vitamins—Friends or Foe?

*...I am the light of the world. He who follows Me shall not walk in darkness,
but have the light of life* (John 8:12).

Jesus said in God's Word, *"I am the light of the world."* He was very vocal in pointing out righteous principles. I want to expand your mindset. Hippocrates said in 400 BC, "Let food be your medicine and let medicine be your food." I have used supplementation in my practice from the beginning. Generally, patients come to my office for my opinion about how they can achieve a greater level of health. Due to ignorance of facts or a false sense of security from reading a magazine article, consumers purchase a lot of bottles of various products. Not all of the products are wrong, but if the products they were taking helped, would they be at my door step?

Synthetic, fractionalized supplements from questionable sources can actually create a toxic state in an already weakened body. Let's talk and think: One orange generally has twenty-five milligrams of whole complex C. Eating more than two, or fifty milligrams of vitamin C, will result in digestive distress. Is five hundred milligrams of synthetic ascorbic acid vitamin C safe? I do not take vitamin C. I do not bruise easily, and my bumps and cuts heal in a timely fashion. I want you to focus on whole food, organic raw vegetables and fruit. I focus on whole food. I strongly encourage my patients to use whole food, cold processed, low dosage supplements versus high potency, synthetic products. Synthetic, higher dosage protocols are best for a short time. You need to modify your lifestyle for optimal health.

Natural Prescription for Health: Add one whole food, raw organic vegetable to your daily diet this week.

Personal Thoughts/Goals:

_____

_____

_____

_____

Day 317

Fix it! Don't Patch it!

No one sews a piece of unshrunk cloth on an old garment;
or else the new piece pulls away from the old... (Mark 2:21).

Jesus was talking to His followers about restoration by telling them the story of the patch and wineskin. This prompts me to tell you about cholesterol. Cholesterol is not bad or good. It was created to have a very important purpose. Low density lipid (LDL) is the carrier that has been instructed to take cholesterol to the site of inflammation or injury so cell membranes can still function. High density lipid (HDL) is the carrier that takes cholesterol back to the liver.

Think of cholesterol as a firefighter. Firefighters put out fires; therefore, cholesterol is a friend of the body—probably news to you. LDL, in all fairness, is doing its job by attempting to put out the fire. This is important, and it is the opposite of what we are generally told. Cholesterol-lowering drugs literally destroy the good guys, or firemen. Sugar, dairy, heavy use of saturated fat with arachidonic acid and trans fat (margarine), excessive Omega 6 fat use, stress and insulin, alcohol, and smoking create inflammation. Stop the inflammation and LDL goes home. This is good news!

Natural Prescription for Health: Inflammation caused by eating sugar, insulin, trans fat, and dairy *creates* a body response of LDL cholesterol elevation. Avoid these substances.

Personal Thoughts/Goals:

_____

_____

_____

_____

Day 318

Dairy and Pain

Get wisdom! Get understanding! (Proverbs 4:5).

The people of Israel were to relocate to the land flowing with milk and honey. It has currently been estimated that up to one-third of the world population is now sensitive to cow's milk. Milk has a fat in its structure called arachidonic acid. This particular fat creates pain. I have many patients who are literally addicted to milk with relentless sinus, hand, back, hip, ankle, and head pain (basically pain anywhere). We *always* see improvement in their conditions when milk is eliminated or minimized. Chronic ear and sinus infections leave within days.

If you crave milk, add sesame seeds and almonds to your oatmeal and salads. Substitute flax and black currant oils for the fat cravings and chicken, turkey, or fish to satisfy your protein need. Your pain will happily subside if milk is the cause.

Natural Prescription for Health: Do you have pain without cause? Add sesame seeds, almonds, and mixed greens to your diet while eliminating dairy for one month.

Personal Thoughts/Goals:

_____

_____

_____

_____

Day 319

The Fountain of Renewed Youth

Then I will sprinkle clean water on you, and you shall be clean (Ezekiel 36:25).

The thought of agelessness has motivated people since the curse. Billions of dollars are spent—*"so that your youth is renewed like the eagle's"* (Ps. 103:5)—on hair coloring, cosmetic dentistry, and surgery—straightening, lifting, tucking, and removing.

Stimulating tissue restoration at the cellular level from "the inside out" is a foundational principal that is simple to do. Clean machines work better. Skin complexion will glow by consuming water from a pure source. Water hydrates cells, promoting elimination of toxins and "free radicals" damage (browning of an apple, oxidation). Toxic relief minimizes strain on body-releasing nutrients for restoration and repair versus existence. Drinking water will stimulate bowel elimination, relieve chronic sinusitis, and even improve toxins released while breathing. Your body can focus on rejuvenation for your renewed youthful spirit.

Natural Prescription for Health: Add midmorning and afternoon vegetable snacks instead of cookies, crackers, or candy bars.

Personal Thoughts/Goals:

_____

_____

_____

_____

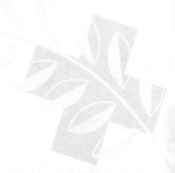

Day 320

Your Hairs Are Counted

But the very hairs on your head are all numbered... (Luke 12:7).

Jesus mentioned in the Word that God knows the number of hairs on your head. Did you ever try to count hairs? You might get to seventy-five. Hair is on the crown of your head and potentially over most of your body. Hair has many purposes. It conserves body heat, protects the scalp, and is a part of the sensory system. The hair shaft is the part that grows above the skin surface. It is alive and is affected by hormones, enzymes, blood, perspiration, environment, and genetics. What you apply to your hair can be absorbed into the body. Lead-based ingredients can be especially harmful. Hair quality, amount, and texture are affected by your dietary choices.

Hair tissue analysis reveals much about your current body health. Toxins and minerals are more concentrated in the hair. I see patterns and ratios that help me determine potential body dysfunction. High copper levels are often seen with low zinc. This pattern is common in females with high estrogen and men with prostate enlargement. Evaluating hair can assist in altering lifestyle patterns.

Natural Prescription for Health: Eat mineral-rich organic greens raw, steamed, or sautéed; kale, asparagus, celery, green beans, and peas are excellent sources of minerals. Be creative with your green foods. Hair strength, quality, and thicknesses are related to gland function and mineral levels.

Personal Thoughts/Goals:

_____

_____

_____

_____

Day 321

Keep Good Company

...He, the Spirit of truth...will guide you into all truth... (John 16:13).

Do you like what you see and hear about yourself? This may seem like an elementary question, but it is real. Are you happy? If not, why not? It has been researched that it takes twenty-one days to develop a new pattern. First Corinthians 15:33 says, *"Do not be deceived: 'Evil company corrupts good habits.'"* Who do you hang around with? Basic good habits like reading and mediating on the Word daily *"...will make your way prosperous and then you will have good success"* (Josh. 1:8). This is true regardless of age—young, intermediate, or advanced. *"...Those who seek the Lord shall not lack any good thing"* (Ps. 34:10).

It is my desire for you to develop the habit of optimal health. Seek and find an accountability partner. When two or more are gathered in His name, He will be there in the midst of them. I pray for you to have another friend—the Holy Spirit.

Natural Prescription for Health: Start every day with a mid or low glycemic breakfast. Avoid pastries and items that will initiate refined carbohydrate cravings all day. Revisit pattern two—Breakfast.

Personal Thoughts/Goals:

_____

_____

_____

_____

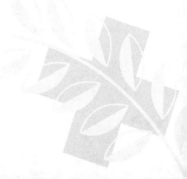

Day 322

Fiber Up

Whole-grain fiber may slow artery clogging, according to a study of more than two hundred postmenopausal women with heart disease.

Angiograms showed slower artery clogging over three years in women who consumed more than six servings of whole grains per week or in women who ate at least three grams of fiber from whole grains for every one thousand calories they consumed each day.

What to do? This kind of study cannot prove that whole grains slow down artery clogging, but it's one more reason to switch to whole-grain breads, cereals, crackers, rice, pasta, cookies, and so forth. You may want to consider no sugar, gluten-free, and potato starch-free items.[57]

> When I first came to see Dr. Bob, I had joint pain and a loss of mobility in my left femoral joint. I was also taking antidepressants, birth control, and muscle relaxants. Following Dr. Bob's advice, I have greatly decreased my sugar intake. I consume little or no soda, ice cream, candy, or cakes, and I avoid fast food restaurants. Eliminating sugar and processed foods while switching to organic foods as well as eating a beet daily has been difficult. However, since making these lifestyle changes, I am no longer on medications, and I no longer suffer with PMS, depression, or muscle spasms. I also have increased mobility. I am so grateful for the treatment I have received. I am hopeful that I will keep my health and mobility while preventing any chronic illnesses.
> —Dody Cuson

Personal Thoughts/Goals:

_____

_____

_____

_____

Day 323

Jesus the Businessman

After these things, the Lord appointed seventy others also, and sent them two by two before His face into every city and place where He himself was about to go (Luke 10:1).

The premise of this optimal health devotional guide is about learning and acting. Jesus was a spiritual leader as well as an astute business leader. He chose a variety of individuals to train to be His master workers and three special followers to be in His inner circle. Jesus Himself was in constant communication with His CEO, His Father. Jesus took the time to pray, eat, and rest. He continuously taught His inner circle of master workers and followers. The disciples surprisingly did not always act in faith on the principles they were learning. Jesus also went to the people; He was not stationary. He spoke in simple terms and spoke with confidence and authority. He put into action what He was teaching at the time. He told Peter to drop the nets into the water at a different level and they caught a huge number of fish. He created the finest wine, served His own followers, and confronted opposition. Jesus had compassion and helped those in need. His needs were met, and He had overflow.

Natural Prescription for Health: The Word of God is your business manual to tend to God's Kingdom. Read the Gospels—Matthew, Mark, Luke, and John.

Personal Thoughts/Goals:

_____

_____

_____

_____

Day 324

The "Itis" Family

Thus, I will bless you while I live; I will lift up my hands in Your name (Psalm 63:4).

You know the family names: bursitis, arthritis, tendonitis. Tissue names with an -*itis* at the end usually mean "inflammation of." A common problem, especially for females in their late thirties and early forties, is bursitis. Bursitis prevents and even stops a person's ability to raise their arms and hands. Satan will do whatever he can to keep you from praising the Lord by raising your hands in worship.

This is what I see as a common cause of bursitis. The patient has a pH state (acid or alkaline) of being alkaline, like baking soda. I strongly encourage no citrus—oranges, grapefruit, or tangerines, either the juice or the fruit itself. Citrus creates an alkaline state in the body.

Splash organic apple cider vinegar on your salad. Take up to 150 milligrams of a whole food source of B6 a day, which helps eliminate inflammation. A digestive aide with Betaine HCL is also useful in stabilizing your pH. Go ahead and raise those hands!

Natural Prescription for Health: Replace fresh and commercial citrus juice with eight ounces of homemade carrot, apple, cucumber, beet, ginger, celery, and parsley juice.

Personal Thoughts/Goals:

_____

_____

_____

_____

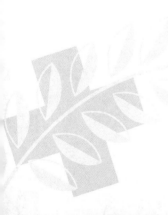

Day 325

Eyes—Windows to the Soul

You hold my eyelids open... (Psalm 77:4).

God created the body to be an interdependent unit working together for one common purpose, just as He created the Church Body for one purpose. Visions, seeing with your mind's eye as Jacob did in Genesis 31:11, are a direct connection to the throne room.

Are you bothered by spots or floaters in front of your eyes? Commonly called vitreous floaters, these annoying events are often self-correcting by adding one organic raw carrot, chopped or grated, on your mixed green salad. Overworked and stressed livers are the storage house of the fat soluble vitamin A that is critical for proper eye health. Minimize toxic foods and beverages that promote liver stress. Have your healthcare physician rule out any other cause for peace of mind. And then enjoy your new level of health.

Natural Prescription for Health: Slice carrots into your mixed green salad.

Personal Thoughts/Goals:

_____

_____

_____

_____

Day 326

You Eat What You Speak

A man's stomach shall be satisfied from the fruit of his mouth;
from the produce of his lips he shall be filled (Proverbs 18:20).

Are you happy with your lot in life? Physically, your stomach is filled with items that you purchase. Your ability to create income is directly related to the words you speak. When was the last time you took an extended learning program to increase your ability to communicate? Skill sets need to be sharp. The problems you solve in life impact your financial well-being.

I would encourage you to read God's Word daily. Speak life-enhancing words. Communicate with love. Think before you speak! Say uplifting comments to all.

Now, when it comes to eating—have you ever thought about leaving the table a little hungry? Do you *need* seconds? Avoid bread with meals. Do not end a meal with dessert. Eating while in distress creates poor digestion. Always eat slowly and drink a small amount of fluids with your meals.

Natural Prescription for Health: Eat and chew slowly. Do not eat while in emotional distress.

Personal Thoughts/Goals:

_____

_____

_____

_____

Day 327

Silver Hair

The silver-haired head is a crown of glory,
if it is found in the way of righteousness (Proverbs 16:31).

Do you have gray or silver hair? Are you also tired and low on energy? Let me share with you what I have learned through mineral tissue hair analysis. The cause of gray hair is chronic fatigue—exhaustion. It is nature's way of warning us that we are running out of energy. It is the minerals in your body that give hair its color. It is true that some people with gray hair have a great deal of energy. What these people don't realize is that they are maintaining their energy levels by using up mineral reserves that are not supposed to be touched. This is why their hair is gray and not dark.

Black hair gets its color from the minerals manganese and iron. Manganese and iron are two minerals your cells need to produce energy. People who are exhausted have depleted minerals. Calcium and zinc usually deposit in your hair as you become exhausted. The process is gradual. People tend to slow as they lose minerals. The body goes into slow oxidation. Overnight gray or white hair can occur when someone experiences a major shock or stress. The good news is it can be reversed. Artificially coloring your hair does not get to the cause of the problem.

Natural Prescription for Health: Gray hair covered with coloring? Try a mineral-rich unrefined salt, nuts, or organic greens.

Personal Thoughts/Goals:

_____

_____

_____

_____

Day 328

Strengthen the Hands

Therefore strengthen the hands which hang down... (Hebrews 12:12).

God has us in His hand. We are the work of God's hands. Jesus placed His hands on people. Hands with an opposable thumb allow dexterity and manipulation of tools. Hand integrity and strength requires proper input from the neck-based nerve roots. Pain in both hands from carpal tunnel can be caused by decayed discs in the neck, misaligned vertebrae, and poor posture. Thumb pain may be caused by joint inflammation and is helped with 150 milligrams of vitamin B6 daily. Vitamin B6 is also beneficial in relieving a condition in hand tendons called trigger finger. Small deposits develop in tendon finger sleeves on the palm aspect of the hand and actually may need to be snapped into place. The nodules can be tender. B6 is needed to reduce inflammation.

I use Burt's Bee cream on my finger tips for moisture and to prevent painful cuticle cracks. Arthritic nodules reduce by minimizing wheat and dairy products. I have seen severe hand pain leave by eliminating all dairy products.

Natural Prescription for Health: Soaking your hand in warm Epsom salt is a source of soothing minerals.

Personal Thoughts/Goals:

_____

_____

_____

_____

Day 329

Caffeine and Parkinson's Disease

Caffeine may lower the risk of Parkinson's disease, say researchers at the US Department of Veterans Affairs in Honolulu.

Robert Abbott and colleagues studied more than eight thousand Hawaiian men of Japanese ancestry who were asked about their diets when they entered the Honolulu Heart Program in the mid-1960s and again in the early 1970s.

Over the next thirty years, 102 of the men were diagnosed with Parkinson's disease. Those who drank no coffee had a two to three times greater risk of Parkinson's than coffee drinkers. Caffeine from other foods was also linked to a lower risk of the disease, but coffee was the largest source of caffeine among the men.

While caffeine is the cause of many health problems, this connection with Parkinson's is interesting. "People who have a predisposition to Parkinson's or early stages of the disease may have a dislike for coffee," says Abbott. "Or, caffeine may delay the degeneration of neurons in the brain." The loss of neurons that produce the neurotransmitter dopamine causes the tremors and other symptoms of Parkinson's.[58]

I had been experiencing severe headaches every day. Due to Dr. DeMaria's advice, I decided to take a serious look at my health issues and take action to correct my problems. Changing my eating habits was a big part of my lifestyle modifications. Dr. DeMaria also helped me understand why I was in so much pain. He was the third healthcare provider that I had been to but the first to accurately diagnose my problem. —Nicole LeMar

Personal Thoughts/Goals:

_____

_____

_____

_____

Day 330

Incline Your Ear to My "Tips"

My son, give attention to my words (Proverbs 4:20).

In order for you to get what you have never had before, you must do what you have never done before. Read, study, and mediate on the Word of God daily. Talk about it with your spouse, parent, friend, or coworker.

What are you learning from the diet and personal journal? Where should you start? Do not throw any food away. Eat the items you have, and slowly add products without trans fat and sugar. Do not make immediate family changes. Go slowly. Drink more water. Eat whole foods, organic preferred. Stay away from trans fat and sugar. Limit snacks to real food. Limit coffee drinking to the morning. Start some type of regular exercise thirty minutes each day. Watch less TV and spend more time with your family. Attend a church community that believes Jesus is the Son of God. Write at least one thank you note each week. Say uplifting, edifying words—or do not speak at all.

Natural Prescription for Health: Commit to reading one self-improvement health book monthly.

Personal Thoughts/Goals:

_____

_____

_____

_____

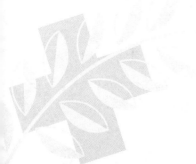

Day 331

An Apple a Day

Like an apple tree among the trees of the woods, so is my beloved among the sons.
I sat down in his shade with great delight, and his fruit was sweet to my taste
(Song of Solomon 2:3).

"*A word fitly spoke is like apples of gold*" (Prov. 25:11). The apple—the not-so-forbidden-fruit—from Bible passages to Newton's Law of Physics breakthroughs, has starred throughout history. New research has uncovered what may be the apple's most enduring role to date: protecting the brain and colon from disease. Quercetin is an antioxidant (stops rust) that appears to be better than vitamin C at shielding test animal brain cells from oxidative (rust) damage. This damage leads to Alzheimer's and other brain dementias. Fresh, organic apples, especially the skins, are a great source of quercetin.

Another compound called procyanidins found in the flesh and skin of apples reduced the amount of colon tumors in laboratory animals. All apples have procyanidins, but apples that taste a little acidic have more. I encourage my patients to eat at least half an apple daily.

Natural Prescription for Health: Thinly sliced apples added to your mixed green salad satisfy the desire for sweets.

Personal Thoughts/Goals:

_____

_____

_____

_____

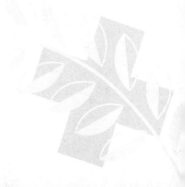

Day 332

Away With Stiff Necks

...Do not speak with a stiff neck (Psalm 75:5).

Did you wake this morning with a stiff left neck and shoulder area pain—again? My evidence-based experience suggests that the most common cause of the relentless, gnawing, chronic pain is precipitated by an internal organ referral.

Sweet and dried fruits, including but not limited to raisins, bananas, grapes, figs, apricots, and pineapple, as well as sugar-based items, always aggravate the left neck. Dairy products, especially those with sugar ingredients, can also create nagging pain. Why? Clinically it is referred via a visceral (organ) somatic (skin) circuit loop.

Malachi 3:10 says, *"And try Me now on this...."* Eliminate these food items for one week. Then add your favorite and wait to see what happens. The results will be life-changing—I've seen it happen many times for my patients.

Natural Prescription for Health: Avoid bananas, raisins, grapes, pineapple, dairy, and sugar if you suffer with chronic neck pain.

Personal Thoughts/Goals:

_____

_____

_____

_____

Day 333

Who Heals All Diseases

…Who heals all your diseases (Psalm 103:3).

We are so blessed that our Heavenly Father put the greatest healer of all inside of us—Himself. I pray wisdom for all of you to understand that satan stole something from humankind in the Garden. Even nature (see Rom. 8:19) eagerly waits for restoration.

See yourself healthy. Speak to your body happy, health-promoting statements. Do not say you have your "normal summer cold or winter pneumonia." Jesus set us free from the bondage of satan. Your body sends messages over a layer of fat on nerves called the myelin sheath. Eat good fat, not human-made fat, regardless of the name or research. Trans fat or partially hydrogenated fat is a poison and interferes with your body's ability to communicate.

Your body is made of three parts—body, mind, and spirit. I pray that your spirit keeps your physical body disease-free. Communicate health—speak life.

Natural Prescription for Health: Say out loud, "I am happy, healthy, and fun to be with!"

Personal Thoughts/Goals:

_____

_____

_____

_____

Day 334

Gall of Bitterness

He has filled me with bitterness, He has made me drink worm wood
(Lamentations 3:15).

Bitterness can evolve into a deep-rooted issue that can destroy human life. Continuous fretting over conversation or unresolved conflict can birth a spirit of bitterness. Practice forgiveness. Become a blessing to someone; you reap what you sow.

In the physical realm, a bitter metal taste in the mouth is a body signal to me of liver/gallbladder distress. Bile is made in the liver. An overworked liver creates thick, sticky, poor quality bile. The liver actually transfers a portion of its duties in filtering to dealing with anger. Feeling melancholy can be translated to black bile. You want free-flowing bile, not inhibition from emotional distress. Certain pharmaceutical companies suggest that aspirin use also causes a bitter taste in the mouth. Aspirin irritates stomach lining with blood loss that can cause digestive distress.

Eat half an apple daily. Drink a cup of hot or cold fresh-squeezed lemon water daily.

Natural Prescription for Health: Gallbladder removed? Add a bovine-sourced bile salt supplement to your daily protocols along with your half apple, beet, and carrot.

Personal Thoughts/Goals:

_____

_____

_____

_____

Day 335

Joint Health

For the word of God is living and powerful...piercing...even to the...joints
(Hebrews 4:12).

Pain paralyzes up to eighty percent of the people in the US. Why do we have so much joint pain? Besides trauma or injury, there are several causes for joint pain. Alignment of a joint is essential for proper mechanics. Alignment is affected by the continual push down of gravity. Neck, back, hip, knee, ankle, and foot alignment is necessary to minimize weight bearing joint pain. But clinically I have seen some of the most distorted, twisted bodies not have any pain.

"Why?" you might be thinking. The answer: "I have had pain my whole life. I can't remember a day without taking a pain reliever." Prescription pain medications or remedies right off the shelf put stress on the liver and kidneys and only mask the symptoms of the root cause of pain.

Try this natural remedy. For one month eat or drink no dairy products—dairy does not include eggs. Use unsweetened almond, rice, or coconut milks as a replacement. Month two, minimize sugar. Sugar steals minerals needed to make natural pain relievers. All along, drink water from a pure source. Finally add flax oil, one tablespoon per one hundred pounds of body weight.

Natural Prescription for Health: No dairy products for one month. Journal your typical diet—tomatoes, white potatoes, green pepper, and eggplant can also cause pain. It is possible your pain can be precipitated by sweet fruits; also be aware of gluten. One person's passion may be another's poison.

Personal Thoughts/Goals:

_____

_____

_____

_____

Day 336

Salt and Soda

If people ate less salt, they would need to drink less liquid, including soda, say British researchers. Their studies confirm that the more salt people consume, the more fluid their kidneys excrete, and the thirstier they become. If Americans consumed no more than the recommended 2,400 milligrams of sodium a day, they'd probably drink one less twelve-ounce soda (or other beverage) each day.

"Best known for its Pepsi-Cola soft drinks brand, PepsiCo generates 66 percent of its operating profits from its Frito-Lay snacks business," says report coauthor Graham MacGregor of St. George's Hospital Medical School in London. "This industry has been preeminent in trying to create doubt about the relationship between salt intake and blood pressure, presumably in the hope of protecting its soft drink sales."[59]

Natural Prescription for Health: Cut back on soda, sodium chloride, and salt.

> I had been depressed and nervous. I had problems with my left arm and was
> taking Prozac, Zamis, Efflizer, and Ionipon. Since beginning care with Dr.
> DeMaria, I have stopped taking Prozac and am cutting down on Ionipon.
> I am now taking natural vitamins following Dr.'s recommendations. This has
> helped quite a bit, but has taken a bit of time for me. People should pray
> about not taking any medication or at least cut down gradually, then quit.
> —Heidi Galauner

Personal Thoughts/Goals:

_____

_____

_____

_____

Time for Him

Let's face it; we live in a very compressed time frame. Our minutes are constantly divided between family, friends, career, and coworkers. Are you taking regular time to be with your Maker? Jesus prayed and communicated with his Heavenly Father on an ongoing level. You can have a consciousness of prayer during daily routine. Form the pattern of speaking to God. He lives in you. He is omnipresent. Schedule God-time into every day. He will never leave you. Take time to listen to Him. The Holy Spirit, the Comforter, is always with you—talk to Him, listen for Him. One of my many favorite verses in the Bible includes John 16:13—let the Holy Spirit speak to your spirit and guide your daily activities.

The Bible is your guide to a God-filled life. It is not doing you any good just sitting on your coffee table. Open it during the down and scheduled times in your life. I combine Word and prayer time in the morning. You don't need to speed through; go slowly, stop, listen, and act on what you are meditating on. Regular Word time will create a mindset of godly presence. My suggestion for this new pattern is to have a specific time in the day to read God's Word. Try reading it out loud. You'll be blessed.

Day 337

Lengthen Your Days

The days of his youth You have shortened... (Psalm 89:45).

Biblical principles, when followed, promote health. Patterns of life lay the foundation for life. What you think about yourself molds your life at any age. Thoughts prompt action. Positive action develops into healthy habits. You can compromise your effectiveness while you are on the earth by choosing unhealthy, destructive habits.

Do you say uplifting comments to your loved ones? Your current emotional and physical state is directly related to what you speak. What are you feeding your spirit? How much time are you being entertained by television?

You can improve who you will be in the next five years by taking two steps: meet new people and read more books. My wife and I pray for new Christian, God-loving individuals to enter our lives. We enjoy reading God-inspired books to fill our minds. Reading opens a whole new world. We do not participate in risky behavior or worldly destructive patterns.

Natural Prescription for Health: Intentionally pray for new people to enter your life.

Personal Thoughts/Goals:

_____

_____

_____

_____

Day 338

What You See Is What You Get

Then the Angel of God spoke to me in a dream saying…. "Lift your eyes now and see, that all the rams which leap on the flocks are streaked, speckled, and gray-spotted…"
(Genesis 31:11-12).

Jacob was an interesting character in the Bible. He had favor on his life and communicated with the Lord. God saw something in him. One of my favorite events in Jacob's life is how he was able to take the vision from the Lord and turn it into increase. Laban, Jacob's father-in-law, was favored because of Jacob. They both attempted to outwit each other. Jacob peeled the bark from trees so that the bark appeared spotted. He chose the healthiest animals from the flock, and while they were mating, he placed the speckled branches in their sight. His flock grew and was separate from Laban's. He was very industrious, and the finances generated from the event created wealth for the twelve tribes. (See Genesis 31.)

God has a plan for everyone's life. It is your responsibility to seek the Lord in your *daily* quiet time. What vision has the Lord given to you about your health in the last several months? Do you have clothes in your closet that used to fit, but now they are too big because you are following the guide to optimal health? What further steps need to be taken to reach your health goals? How can you become the instrument God created you to be spiritually, physically, and emotionally?

Natural Prescription for Health: What is the Lord showing you today? Don't wait—act!

Personal Thoughts/Goals:

_____

_____

_____

_____

Day 339

You Are Not a Grasshopper

*There we saw the giants…and we were like grasshoppers in our own sight,
and so we were in their sight* (Numbers 13:33).

The Lord wants us to *"prosper in all things and be in* [good] *health…"* (3 John 2). What would the world be like today if Christopher Columbus, an experienced sea navigator, would have listened to the educated land lovers? Columbus overcame fear. God was his navigator. According to the memoirs and legend of Columbus, the Holy Spirit directed his course.

You need to be like Columbus, Joshua, and Caleb. Are you looking at an unfriendly health circumstance or issue? The power that made the body can heal the body. Do not succumb to fear. First, you will need to change lifestyle patterns. Do not expect new results with old patterns. Eat less processed food. Focus on detoxifying by drinking more water and eating raw or baked beets. Do not be intimidated by a medical report. Draw a line in the sand and make a decision to do something.

Natural Prescription for Health: Love is the mother of faith. Faith casts out fear. What lifestyle pattern needs to be changed and/or eliminated?

Personal Thoughts/Goals:

_____

_____

_____

_____

Day 340

Life Is in the Blood

And He [the Lord] *said, "What have you done? The voice of your brother's blood cries out to Me from the ground"* (Genesis 4:10).

Blood talks. You might not literally hear it, but a skilled clinician can tell you a lot about yourself just by examining the blood drawn from a pin prick. The blood of Abel cries out today. Blood is so important. The blood of Jesus was poured out for us. Covenant is based on blood.

Pink, or light, shades of blood indicate your blood is not carrying enough iron, which means a lack of oxygen. Oxygen is necessary for life. Thin, liquid blood is the result of too much aspirin, blood thinners, and overdoing fish oils. Do not be duped by getting blood too thin; this could cause internal bleeding and even strokes. Have your bleeding time checked. Heavy menstrual flow associated with elevated estrogen, dark tar blood in the stool, red blood from the rectal irritation or colon problems must be addressed as the source of poor blood conditions.

Eat a variety of foods to feed the body, which creates blood. Mixed greens are an excellent source of chlorophyll and vitamin K and magnesium. An alternative source of iron is from an herb called yellow dock. Your life is dependent on the quality of your blood.

Natural Prescription for Health: Gluten diets may impair iron metabolism, creating a chronic anemic condition causing fatigue.

Personal Thoughts/Goals:

_____

_____

_____

_____

Day 341

Music to My Ears—Worship

Then David and all Israel played music before God with all their might, with singing, on harps, on stringed instruments, on tambourines, on cymbals, and with trumpets (1 Chronicles 13:8).

Hearing the Word of God increases faith. Hearing is one of the five senses that is written literally and figuratively about throughout the New Testament. Jesus was always telling people that they have ears to hear and charging them to pay attention. Music to God's ears is worship. I know there are many forms of worship. God is Spirit; we are to worship Him in spirit and truth. Saul had an annoying spirit that was relieved by David playing the harp or lyre, soothing music to his ears. Music, musical instruments, and worship were also used offensively in Israel's battles against the enemy.

People can be calmed by music. Music can soothe the nervous system, calm your physiology—or music can be irritating. Feed your emotions. Sing worship melodies to calm the storms of life. David praised the Lord until he was exhausted when the tabernacle returned.

Natural Prescription for Health: While on the go, listening to praise and worship music on your preferred audio equipment will enhance your relationship with the Lord.

Personal Thoughts/Goals:

_____

_____

_____

_____

Day 342

Bitterness—A Life Zapper

Pursue peace with all people…lest any root of bitterness springing up cause trouble…
(Hebrews 12:14-15).

The Lord knows bitterness is a poison and will cause trouble. In his book, *Your Liver, Your Lifeline,* Dr. Jack Tips succinctly discusses the enormous role the liver plays in our daily function. Optimal physical, emotional, and chemical health depends on all the body systems functioning at their peak performance.

Perpetual feelings of bitterness can destroy a person in record time. Liver function is not only affected by what you eat and breathe, but it also responds to emotions. Bitterness over any matter stops the liver from completing its job description for detoxification. It literally retools itself to create the nutrients to handle and deal with your emotional stress.

Do you have an issue with someone or something? You can watch your diet, exercise, not smoke or drink alcohol, and still have sickness or even premature death if you harbor bitterness. Jesus told us to forgive seventy times seventy, which is a lot!

Natural Prescription for Health: Forgive and forget as far as the East is from the West any and all who have offended you.

Personal Thoughts/Goals:

_____

_____

_____

_____

Day 343

Ducking Diabetes

Weight loss and exercise prevent diabetes more effectively than drugs, says a study of more than three thousand overweight, middle-aged people who had higher-than-normal blood sugar (but not diabetes).

Each got either a placebo, Glucophage (a drug used to treat high blood sugar), or sixteen one-on-one sessions to help them lose weight and exercise. After nearly three years, twenty-nine percent of the people in the placebo group had developed diabetes, compared with twenty-two percent of the Glucophage takers and just fourteen percent of those in the exercise-and-weight-loss group.

The exercisers didn't need to run marathons. Roughly fifty-eight percent of them met the exercise goal (at least two and a half hours a week of moderate aerobic activity like brisk walking). And thirty-eight percent met the weight-loss goal (they dropped at least seven percent of their body weight by eating a healthy low-calorie, low-fat diet).[60]

Natural Prescription for Health: Get off the couch, office chair, or driver's seat for at least twenty to thirty minutes of walking or other activity every day. And cut calories with a healthy diet that includes lots of fruits and vegetables.

> When I first came to see Dr. DeMaria, I had terrible back pain. I was also taking medication for high blood pressure and high cholesterol. Following Dr. Bob's advice, I have changed my diet, and I am now exercising, which I couldn't do before coming here. It has been difficult absorbing all the new information, which is quite the opposite of what we are used to hearing. The information and care provided by Dr. Bob has improved my life in every way; just being able to learn why and how things work the way they do and how eating certain foods can help you instead of taking drugs. I look forward to coming here. I am so glad I was guided in this direction. I thank God every day! —Sue Clem

Personal Thoughts/Goals:

_____

_____

_____

_____

Day 344

Open Your Eyes

And Elisha prayed and said, "Lord, I pray open his eyes that he may see" (2 Kings 6:17).

It is time! You have been reading for months now. You should be experiencing great advances in your health. I know that you are thoroughly loving this experience—this optimal health devotional guide was written for you!

Here's the *big* one. God wants His children set free; open your eyes! You choose your level of health existence. Medicine does not cure you. The spirit of life in you heals you! Genesis 2:7 says, *"Then the Lord God formed man of the dust of the ground and breathed into his nostrils the breath* [or spirit] *of life; and man became a living being."* When you breathe, you are breathing God. God created the air we breathe! He created the food we eat.

You make choices. Do you choose human-made mutated, chemically altered, toxic foods and beverages? Stop it! Stop it now! Eat whole food and drink pure water. Read God's Word and meditate on Psalm 1:2—chew on it! Get wisdom and discipline.

Natural Prescription for Health: Let the Word reveal to you what you need to change for optimal health! First Corinthians 2:14 says, *"But the natural man does not receive the things of the Spirit of God, for they are foolishness to him; nor can he know them, because they are spiritually discerned."*

Personal Thoughts/Goals:

_____

_____

_____

_____

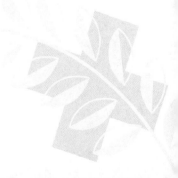

Day 345

Crowd Pleasers

So Pilate, wanting to satisfy the crowd... (Mark 15:15).

Areal challenge I see with individuals today is the perpetual desire to make everyone happy. This can lead to stress, anxiety, and depression. I would like you to incorporate a new way of thinking for your life and to learn how to diplomatically say no. Memorize this statement: "I cannot say yes at this time—no."

People pleasers are always busy, which causes the potential to be consistently below par in the things they are trying to accomplish. Bringing work home from the office and numerous church and community activities can take a toll on already overextended schedules. I believe you should logically participate in activities and be productive in your career—but know when to say no.

Do you get enough sleep? Sleep is the time when your body repairs and maintains itself. Do you spend time meditating and speaking to your Heavenly Father? How much personal and group family time are you enjoying? Do you need to resign from an organization or sell a "toy" that interferes with optimal health time? If you're afraid to say no, remember that you are taking a step to better health—there is no need to feel guilty.

Natural Prescription for Health: Schedule too full to spend time with the family? Learn to politely say, "I cannot say yes at this time."

Personal Thoughts/Goals:

_____

_____

_____

_____

Day 346

"Rabbi, Eat."

And many of the Samaritans, [Mexicans, Asians, Americans, Indians, Europeans, etc.] *of that* [your] *city believed in Him because of the Word of the woman who testified…* (John 4:39).

Jesus said to them,

My food is to do the will of Him who sent me, and to finish His work. Do you not say, "There are still four months and then comes the harvest? Behold, I say to you, lift up your eyes and look at the fields, for they are already white for harvest. He who reaps receives wages, and gathers fruit for eternal life, that both he who sows and he who reaps may rejoice together" (John 4:34-36).

Food for eternity: harvested souls. We are to be fishers of people.

Natural Prescription for Health: Plant seed (Word); water plants (souls). Tell someone about Jesus today!

Personal Thoughts/Goals:

_____

_____

_____

_____

Day 347

Plugged Conduits (Pipes)

*Now the rest of the acts of Hezekiah—all his might, and how he made
a pool and a tunnel and brought water into the city—are they not
all written in the book...* (2 Kings 20:20).

Jerusalem was a stronghold prior to David coming to the scene. Several tribes and kings attempted to overthrow the walled city without success. David's mighty men swam through a conduit pipe in the water system below the gates, opened the gates of the wall, and let David and his army in.

We have conduit pipes in our body system. They are called blood vessels. Some carry blood to the heart and lungs for oxygen refreshment while others return blood to the cells to do their work. A diet focused on foods that raise insulin—pies, cakes, cookies, and desserts—create a state of inflammation. Inflamed vessels require cholesterol to keep the fire under control. Is your cholesterol high? You may want to think twice and say "no thank you" the next time you are offered a tempting dessert. Always read ingredient labels. Your blood system functioning at one hundred percent is vital for a healthy life.

Natural Prescription for Health: Focus on antioxidant rich apples, blueberries, and spinach. Apple slices or celery sticks with almond butter are a spectacular midmorning stabilizer.

Personal Thoughts/Goals:

_____

_____

_____

_____

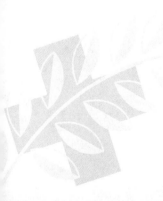

Day 348

My Hero—Caleb

*But My servant Caleb, because he has a different spirit in him
and has followed Me fully, I will bring into the land where he went,
and his descendants shall inherit it* (Numbers 14:24).

Do you have a hero? Who is your mentor? I have several. Martin Luther spoke up and changed the world. Christopher Columbus proved the world was round. Albert Einstein mathematically changed the world's mindset. Caleb had a different spirit. He followed the Lord fully. The Word of God is His manual, His communication tool of love to us. The Ten Commandments, the Books of Leviticus, Numbers, Deuteronomy, Proverbs, and many more, provide insight about how to live a full and healthy God-given life.

Go to your grave empty. Empty out all you have to the Lord. When the other spies along with Caleb saw the giants, what they really saw was the impossibility of the situation. But Caleb did not see himself as inferior. He was with the Lord. The Lord spoke to him. Joshua and Caleb were the only two of the original men who left Egypt to enter the Promised Land. My prayer for you is to see the Lord fully. Read God's Word, and speak the Word. Have a faith mindset. Walk into your promise.

Natural Prescription for Health: Meditate and chew on God's Word daily. Sit quietly and let the Lord speak to you. His words are truly life! Who is your mentor?

Personal Thoughts/Goals:

_____

_____

_____

_____

Day 349

What You *Say* Is What You Get!

My son, give attention to my words; incline your ear to my sayings. Do not let them depart from your eyes; keep them in the midst of your heart; for they are life to those who find them, and health to all their flesh (Proverbs 4:20-22).

God spoke and the earth was created. There is a natural principle called "self-fulfilling prophecy." In other words, when you make statements such as, "I always get pneumonia this time of year," or "I am so clumsy," or "I am so absentminded," you are instructing your brain and nervous system to carry out directions that are not life-promoting. Become aware of the words you are speaking. Avoid at all cost negative comments. Speak life-enhancing statements, *even if you do not feel one hundred percent.* Do not dwell in your own pity party. It may be time to get new friends. Do not purposely be around negative-speaking people. Misery loves company.

You are the temple of the Holy Spirit. I would not watch or read the news on any medium. Continual amusing of yourself by "hibernating" on the Internet is using precious time that could be spent with your family and in the Word. Take time to develop a positive, health-promoting mindset and vocabulary. Read a chapter in the Book of Proverbs daily. Start today.

Natural Prescription for Health: Think before you speak. Remember, you will receive what you speak.

Personal Thoughts/Goals:

_____

_____

_____

_____

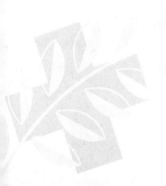

Day 350

Movers and Thinkers

Staying active can help keep your brain in good shape, say two new studies that tracked exercise and mental decline over time.

In the first study that spanned seven years and followed more than 2,200 men who live in Hawaii, aged seventy-one to ninety-three, those who walked the least (less than a quarter mile a day) were nearly twice as likely to be diagnosed with dementia than those who walked the most (more than two miles a day). Men who walked between a quarter and one mile a day had a seventy percent increased risk.

In a second study, which tracked nearly nineteen thousand women, aged seventy to eighty-one, for at least nine years, those who exercised the most had a twenty percent lower risk of cognitive impairment than those who exercised the least. Women who walked for at least one and a half hours a week scored better on memory, attention, and other tests than women who walked less than forty minutes a week.[61]

Natural Prescription for Health: Go for a walk…every day.

I have lung problems (COPD). My lung doctor said I had the worst lungs that he has ever seen. My blood oxygen was only eighty percent. After following Dr. DeMaria's advice, my blood oxygen is now up to ninety percent. I am doing more of my housework. I am thankful Dr. Bob is a Christian and his place of business is blessed by the Lord. —Carol Altman

Personal Thoughts/Goals:

_____

_____

_____

_____

Day 351

Good-bye Gallstones

Being overweight, female, and over forty years of age are some of the classic risk factors for getting gallstones. Spending more than forty hours a week on your fanny may be another, say researchers at the Harvard School of Public Health.

Michael Leitzmann and coworkers followed more than sixty thousand women who had participated in the Nurses' Health Study since 1986. Between 1986 and 1996, 3,257 of the women had surgery to remove a gallstone.

Those who engaged in any exercise for two to three hours a week had about a twenty percent lower risk of gallstone surgery than sedentary women. In contrast, women who spent more than sixty hours a week sitting while at work or in their cars had more than twice the risk of women who spent no more than forty hours a week sitting.

"The risk is slightly elevated from 40 to 60 hours a week of sitting," says Leitzmann, "and really starts to sky-rocket at over 60 hours."[62]

> I brought my daughter, Connor, to see Dr. DeMaria because she was suffering with her asthma. She would be up all night long coughing uncontrollably. She would even miss school the following day. Connor was on her inhaler and nebulizer. The inhaler was causing depression and bouts of crying. It has been difficult, but following Dr. Bob's advice we have limited sugar in our diet and no aspartame. We have added flax oil to our diet. Connor almost never uses her inhaler anymore. Her nebulizer has only been used four times in the last year. Dr. Bob made a health commitment to Connor in 2001. Because of him, we have not been to her pediatrician for her asthma in the last four years.
> —Sherri Csubak

Personal Thoughts/Goals:

_____

_____

_____

_____

Day 352

What Controls Your Spirit?

I say then: Walk in the Spirit, and you shall not fulfill the lust of the flesh
(Galatians 5:16).

There was a time in my life when I was controlled like *"...a mighty man who shouts because of wine"* (Ps. 78:65). The spirit of alcohol had me. I was the *typical* social drinker living a life of denial. The control of alcohol nearly destroyed my life, marriage, and practice. The power of the *Holy Spirit*, through a step of faith and much intercessory prayer by family and friends, released me from alcohol's grip. The instant I was released—never desiring to taste again—I was filled with the wisdom of God. First Kings 3:12 says, "I have given you a wise and understanding heart, Solomon."

My prayer for you is that, *whatever* is prohibiting the Holy Spirit from having total charge in your life—alcohol, drugs, sugar, pornography, or something else—you would be released from that yoke so you can receive a *"wise and understanding heart."*

Natural Prescription for Health: Is there a life pattern that is controlling you and is depleting your life? I pray that you seek Jesus and be released by the power of the Holy Spirit.

Personal Thoughts/Goals:

_____

_____

_____

_____

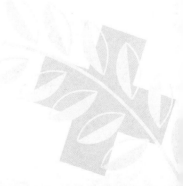

Day 353

Delight the Heart

*Ointment and perfume delight the heart, and the sweetness of
a man's friend gives delight by hearty counsel* (Proverbs 27:9).

Jesus received a gift from the travelers from the East at the beginning of His life. The gifts that He received were both symbolic and practical. Half of the fun in giving is the pleasure the giver has knowing the recipient will have a "feel good" endorphin rush in the brain. God had extreme pleasure giving Jesus to us as a gift—for eternal life.

My suggestion to help your adrenal and stress gland get an injection of "feel good" stimulation is to gift a special someone. Men, flowers always make a great gift; a favorite perfume, one that may bring up positive memories, is always thoughtful. Ladies, men have a favorite dish. Children, young or grown parents love food and companionship. Handwritten thank you notes, a birthday call, any type of unexpected acknowledgment is appreciated by everyone. I am encouraging you to turn it up a notch. The more love and joy you pass on, the greater impact you will make expanding God's Kingdom.

Natural Prescription for Health: Make a call, send a note, buy a gift. Pass on love to one person today.

Personal Thoughts/Goals:

_____

_____

_____

_____

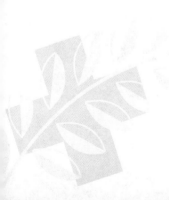

Day 354

See This Truth

And He said to him, "Go, wash in the pool of Siloam"....
So he went and washed, and came back seeing (John 9:7).

Pursue health from the inside out, creating the environment that sharpens "the saw" to live without burnout. The majority of sickness and poor health I treat today is self-inflicted. Again: Poor health is usually self-inflicted. I like to call it death by denial. Your nervous system controls the function of your body. Every tiny cell is directly controlled by this computer system. People are blind to this fact. Correct spinal column alignment with a flow of electrical impulse and healing energy is necessary for optimal health.

I have treated patients with a variety of named conditions. A common one—chronic sinusitis, afflicting up to eighteen percent of the US population—creates billions of dollars for the pharmaceutical industry. I have patients with various histories, including eight sinus drilling procedures with no permanent correction. Correcting a subluxated second cervical neck vertebra, detected by radiography and thermography, releases the power switch, opening the channel from brain cell to tissue cell. Sinus passages can clear in the time it takes to flip a switch. This same sequence of events can be duplicated for any tissue in the body.

Natural Prescription for Health: Do you suffer with chronic poor health? Pray, seek, and locate a skilled spinal adjuster.

Personal Thoughts/Goals:

_____

_____

_____

_____

Day 355

Offensive Favor

Whoever has no rule over his own spirit is like a city broken down, without walls
(Proverbs 25:28).

Discipline is freedom. David trained after he was anointed with oil. He went back to tending sheep. He killed a bear and lion with the help of the Lord. I am sure he practiced with smooth stones in his sling. He no doubt was in optimal physical shape and talented musically. His harp or lyre playing ability soothed Saul's tormented spirit. Music calms the spirit.

What is your capacity? The windows of Heaven are open to us. The Lord wants to bless us. Even a wicked man would not give his son a snake. My suggestion to you is to slow down your life. Find a segment of time daily to read God's Word. Listen to uplifting, positive worship music. The sword of the Spirit is the Word. Your offensive weapon is to study and speak His Word. Speak the Word of God over your health. Do not speak death words—you will ambush your victory. You can't increase the Kingdom of God if you are negative and sick. It is time for a new, clear mindset.

Natural Prescription for Health: Write six items that you are thankful for today. Do that daily for twenty-one days.

Personal Thoughts/Goals:

_____

_____

_____

_____

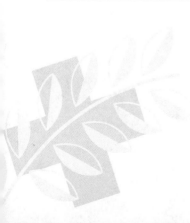

Day 356

Servant's Success Steps

If anyone serves Me, let him follow Me; and where I am, there My servant will be also. If anyone serves Me, him my Father will honor (John 12:26).

Jesus was discussing with His disciples that they were no longer servants, but friends. They were friends partially because of the time spent in His presence. Through learning and role playing, smart, perceptive servants who are well-rewarded will think ahead. We are all servants to someone. In business, CEOs are servants to the board of directors; the board is servant to the shareholders.

Are you happy with how you are treated? If not, or if you want a more productive, happier life—serve more. Send a handwritten thank you to someone who touched you in some way. Fill up your spouse's gas tank without being asked. Take out the garbage or put the newspaper in the recycle bin. Fill up the soap dispenser, or put the new toilet paper roll on the way your spouse prefers. Rake a neighbor's yard. Put flowers on the table. Live a life of giving. God so loved us, He gave His son. To have a friend, be a friend. Ask someone over for a fresh food homemade dinner. Fresh, delicious meals are a special treat.

Natural Prescription for Health: Once a day, do something unexpected to bless someone, no strings attached, no thank you expected.

Personal Thoughts/Goals:

_____

_____

_____

_____

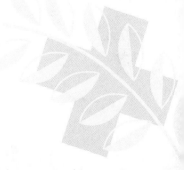

427

Day 357

I Free You This Day

*And now look, I **free** you this day from the chains that were on your hand…. See, all the land* [time] *is before you; wherever it seems good and convenient for you to go, go there* (Jeremiah 40:4, emphasis added).

You are free. You are free! Awesome words. Believers in Jesus are free from sin and death! Throw off the shackles of physical and emotional sickness. You have my permission—I am authorizing you with a renewed warranty on life. You need to follow the Manual for the warranty to remain intact. I know from experience that if you do the following, you will live happy and healthy.

Drink water from a pure source daily. Reverse osmosis is an excellent filter system. A general rule is a half ounce of water per pound of body weight (more cells, need more water). Eat primarily fresh organic vegetables, raw or steamed. Consume protein from an organic source. Focus on chicken, turkey, ocean fish, and lean red meat (no pork). Consume one tablespoon of flax per one hundred pounds of body weight. Avoid refined sugar and all human-made substitutes. *Never* eat trans fat or partially hydrogenated fat. Avoid liver-congesting beverages.

Exercise a minimum of one-half hour daily, weight training and aerobic. Meditate on God's Word constantly. Love everyone. Give to the poor. Have your spine checked for vertebral subluxation. (See John 16:33.) Start a plan to reduce your dependence on medication.

Natural Prescription for Health: Make a quality decision to add one new health pattern to your life per day, week, or month. *Start now!*

Personal Thoughts/Goals:

_____

_____

_____

_____

Day 358

Your Attitude Determines Your Altitude

You were taught with your former way of life, to put off your old self, which is being corrupted by its deceitful desires; to be made new in the attitude of your minds; and to put on the new self… (Ephesians 4:22 NIV).

Jesus was with His disciples for three years, teaching and training them in the way of truth. The Pharisees in the Book of Acts knew the apostles were not formerly trained in the way they were accustomed, and were astonished by the words and confidence that came from Peter's mouth. Peter's mindset was changed. He had a new attitude about Jesus' role in eternal life. He had confidence and boldness to say what was *true*.

You now should have confidence in your understanding of what creates or depletes your own health status. Peter's spiritual growth was experiential in comparison to the world's view of training. You are about to complete your first complete pass through of your health restoration guide. What have you learned?

Your attitude of being proactive about your health should now be grounded in the fact that you have a say in what your health future will be. Take the position now to become what you eat, think, and say. Be a blessing and tell someone.

Natural Prescription for Health: Make a point to review your diet assessment in the breakfast, lunch, and dinner patterns. Are you doing better?

Personal Thoughts/Goals:

_____

_____

_____

_____

Day 359

What Gives Mustard Its Yellow Color?

…The kingdom of heaven is like a mustard seed… (Matthew 13:31).

Mustard seed is a stimulant, diuretic (fluid release), and in large doses, an emetic (causes vomiting). It can be used as a mild laxative and blood purifier, and a tablespoonful acts as a quick emetic.

Externally, the oil is used to stimulate local circulation. A mustard plaster is made by mixing powdered mustard with cold water to make a thick paste. The paste is spread on a cotton cloth. Another thin cloth is placed on the skin and the mustard cloth placed over it. The plaster should remain on the skin until the skin begins to redden and a burning sensation is felt. This is a great technique to improve the movement of fluid in your legs if you feel that there is reduced flow. It will get the blood circulating.

Mustard is one of my favorite condiments; it usually does not contain sugar, as is found in ketchup. The yellow color comes from an herb called tumeric. Tumeric is also a great "anti-tumor" root and can be used as an anti-inflammatory food. Tumeric can be found in the vegetable section of your grocery store.

Natural Prescription for Health: One fourth teaspoon of grated organic tumeric on your mixed green salad two or three times per week would be a logical approach to promote optimal health.

Personal Thoughts/Goals:

_____

_____

_____

_____

430

Day 360

Is There Fungus on Your Toes?

The Lord will strike you with wasting disease, with fever and inflammation, with scorching heat and drought, with blight and mildew, which will plague you all until you perish (Deuteronomy 28:22 NIV).

Your feet are the foundation for your trunk and spinal alignment. Humans are bipeds—we walk on two extremities. In the Old and New Covenant the feet were taken care of with detailed concern. Jesus took the time to wash the disciples' feet as an example of serving. The dusting off of the feet, walking many miles, and sandals that did not wear out are common verses in the Word that describe how important feet were then—and now.

Do you have discolored toe or fingernails? Does your skin itch? Do you have unexplained discomfort that does not appear to respond to treatment? I have recently observed in my practice an unusual number of patients who suffer with chronic fungus issues.

I have discovered in my Natural Health Doctor training that the "seek and destroy" scavengers in your body, called T-lymphocytes, can be inhibited in their activity by elevated levels of hormones from the adrenal gland. The adrenal gland produces more stress hormones when the body is in an "overdrive" condition. Sugar, caffeine, and stimulants can also exaggerate adrenal function resulting in possibly more fungus growth and unchecked bacteria and virus growth.

Natural Prescription for Health: Are you stressed by circumstances that need to be confronted? It is time to say *no* to situations that compromise your health.

Personal Thoughts/Goals:

_____

_____

_____

_____

Day 361

"Âge bien, mon ami": Age Well My Friend

So Methuselah lived 969 years, and he died... (Genesis 5:27 AMP).

In Genesis chapter 5 we're told that one of the oldest men to live on the planet had a child when he was 187 years old. Methuselah went on to have several more children. Now that is aging well wouldn't you say? Caleb was one of the only two original slaves who left Egypt to enter into the Promised Land. He had the same strength and stamina after forty years of wandering that he did when he first saw the large grapes and other food items while on a spying mission.

You can age well. I have seen in my practice that one of the leading causes that promotes longevity is drinking water from a *pure source*. Water bathes cells. Clean machines work better. I have noticed the leading cause of premature aging is smoking cigarettes. The body attempts to clear the toxins entering the lungs because of the smoke and uses precious nutrients to fix damage rather than promote life. Cigarette smokers appear to have drawn, wrinkled skin, a cough, dental implants, veneers, or dentures. Royal jelly, a product of bee hive activity, does help reduce the craving for cigarettes; usually about two thousand milligrams a day is a good start.

Sugar is the next item that stresses the body. Sugar depletes precious minerals and vitamins necessary for cellular function. We live and die at the cellular level. My number one suggestion to promote life is: eat organic whole food every day, especially greens. Eating processed food means the good stuff that decomposes easily and reduces shelf life has been eliminated. Processed food is *dead*. You are what you eat.

Physically exercise a half hour every day. Do something. On an emotional level, don't worry! Be happy. Forgive everyone. Unforgiveness is the root of bitterness.

Natural Prescription for Health: Take a walk and have a laugh today.

Personal Thoughts/Goals:

_____

_____

_____

_____

Day 362

Heart Health

*I call with my whole **heart**; answer me O Lord* (Psalm 119:145 NIV).

Take the time to read Psalm 119. I have many versions of the Bible. One of my favorites is the Personal Promise Bible that I received as a gift from a special friend. In this version, your name replaces personal pronouns in strategic places throughout. Psalm 119 comes alive when your name is inserted. I chose verse 145 that mentions the heart because I want to talk to you about the heart before the year comes to the end.

You accept Jesus into your heart as Lord and Savior to give rebirth to your spirit. In the physical body, I have seen many patients who have had heart distress respond positively to whole food B vitamins. The heart receives electrical impulses like any other muscle in the body. Nerves require B vitamins.

I also have seen patients who have heart distress because their liver is being overworked because they are overweight from overeating. Blood has to flow through the liver before it goes to the heart. A congested liver impedes blood flow. Do you have a large abdomen and varicose or red spider looking veins in your legs? If yes, work on reducing your abdomen; eat more whole foods, including beets, to support the liver. Eat whole grains high in B vitamins, and avoid white bread and snacks—they create heart stress.

Natural Prescription for Health: The herb Dandelion root promotes liver health. Hawthorn berry supports heart function. Talk to your doctor before you make dietary changes.

Personal Thoughts/Goals:

_____

_____

_____

_____

Day 363

No More Pain!

*News about him spread all over Syria, and people brought to him all who were ill with various diseases, those suffering severe **pain**…and he healed them*
(Matthew 4:24 NIV, emphasis added).

Jesus came to set us *free* from the pain of sin and death. He went around on foot healing people of their infirmities. Do you suffer with pain? In my practice, by far the leading reason patients come in is because of some type of pain. I am sure that your pain level is now diminished since beginning this program. Why? Because what you eat can either cause or eliminate pain.

Be aware that pain medication does not correct the reason that your body has pain. Generally, medication designed to relieve pain is fooling Mother Nature. Do you know that your body needs to recognize pain for you to heal? Think about this: Pain is a signal to your brain to send the right nutrients and components to repair. If there is a diminished signal reaching the brain about the pain level, will your body know what to do? I have patients who have taken pain medications for years without improvement before coming into my office. You need to find the *cause* of the pain.

In our practice, we have patients journal (keep track of) their food intake. The following items are the most common that I have seen that cause pain—sugar, dairy, and trans fat. These three are the leaders because they interfere with a pain-relieving fat (tissue hormone that relieves pain and inflammation) called prostaglandin 3. Wheat, citrus, tomatoes, potatoes, green peppers, and eggplant can cause pain in some individuals. Now I am not saying that these foods are bad, but they can be a precipitating factor for some. The most common gnawing cause of mid-back pain from my experience is white potatoes. Sweet fruits, unknown to most, also cause pain and inflammation in the body. I recently had a patient who was drinking nut milk that had sugar in it that caused her pain.

Natural Prescription for Health: Do you suffer with chronic pain? If yes, journal your diet, check for pain food patterns, and delete the ones that are causing the problem. Stealth foods may be the ones you have a passion for; undigested protein particles can create an alarm in the body that you are under attack—endorphins are released and the battle goes on! I would be aware of the following foods that may create pain—gluten foods including wheat, oats, barley, and rye. Also just a gentle reminder some of the most addictive foods can be the cause of your pain. The nightshades, including white potatoes, tomatoes, green pepper, hot peppers, paprika, and eggplant have a chemical in their makeup that, from my clinical experience, creates distress when one has a compromised or congested liver. The nightshades have nicotine in the cell structure and are quite addictive; when was the last time you only ate one potato chip?

Personal Thoughts/Goals:

_____

_____

_____

_____

Day 364

Herbs for Life

*Then God said, "I give you every seed-bearing plant on the face of the whole earth and every tree that has fruit with seed in it. **They will be yours for food**"*
(Genesis 1:29 NIV, emphasis added).

Our Heavenly Father has taken care of us from the very beginning. He has supplied us with food—food to nourish us. I have some herbs that are my favorites. There are many herbs available. Herbs are foods that will stimulate, tonify, sedate, and protect you at the cellular level. You cannot eat indiscriminately and expect the herbs to save you from disease. Be sensible.

The following list of herbs will help you make healthy decisions about herbal intake:

- **Yellow Dock:** liver support and skin health; source of iron

- **Kelp:** source of iodine, vitamins, and minerals; lowers blood pressure

- **Alfalfa:** source of calcium and other minerals

- **Dandelion root/leaf:** liver and kidney purifier

- **Peppermint leaf:** digestive aid, antimicrobial, relieves flu symptoms

- **Hawthorn berry:** heart health and stamina

- **Black cohosh:** female tonic and lowers blood pressure

- **Gymnema:** takes away the craving for sweets

- **Chaste tree:** female organ support, promotes progesterone

- **Collosonia root:** aids hemorrhoids and varicose veins

- **Licorice:** stimulates the entire system

Natural Prescription for Health: I would encourage you to choose herbs from an organic source. Kelp is one of the world's greatest food sources, but because we have polluted the planet so much, the constituency of kelp has been compromised.

Personal Thoughts/Goals:

_____

_____

_____

_____

Day 365

Be a Blessing Every Day!

And He led them out as far as Bethany, and He lifted up His hands and blessed them. Now it came to pass, while He blessed them, that He was parted from them and carried up into heaven (Luke 24:50).

WOW! That must have been a sight, seeing Jesus leave! I have heard it preached that it is grander to receive blessings than it is to need a miracle. Jesus blessed meals and the people who followed Him, including the children.

Deb, my wife, and I were so touched by the way Jesus left the planet that we decided to create an entity named Bethany Blessing Ministry. One of the primary purposes of this nonprofit organization is to assist missionaries when they are home on furlough. We would love to have you partner with us. A portion of the profit from each of these books sold is used to purchase houses needed in the ministry.

I was blessed by God to share this healthy living information with you. It amazes me when I reread the pages how blessed I really am. I suggest you look for blessings in your life. If you do not expect or look for them, you may not find them. I have patients tell me every day how blessed they have been to learn that they can have an impact on their own lives. I am glad that you finished the book, and pray that you pass on what you have learned. If I don't see you here on earth…look for me in Heaven.

Natural Prescription for Health: To gain a friend is to be a friend. Bless someone today in an extraordinarily positive way.

Personal Thoughts/Goals:

_____

_____

_____

_____

Congratulations!

You, and your inner support circle of family and friends have made it through the last twelve months learning how to have optimal health—and I am excited for you!

I look forward to your comments about how your life has been impacted and changed to one of optimal health.

—Sincerely, Dr. Bob

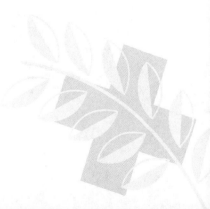

Relationship Renewal

Now you have an opportunity to change your eternal destiny. The Bible is not a story book. It is our Heavenly Father's communication tool to us—our "Instant Messenger." God is Spirit. We are to worship Him in spirit and truth.

When we are born, our natural spirits that reside in our clay bodies, are dead to the things of God. The natural person thinks God things are foolish. You cannot see the Kingdom of God unless your spirit is reborn.

By reading the Book of Romans chapter 10, verses 9 and 10, you can kindle your spirit by making Jesus the Lord of your life, as I did many years ago. It says in the Word that if you recognize you are a sinner, which we all are, and say in your heart (mind) that you would like Jesus to reside in you and become the Lord of your life, you will be saved. Saved from what, you ask? Eternal separation from God upon the death of your physical body. Make the commitment to Jesus now—ask for forgiveness and accept His love. Next, tell somebody about your commitment—speaking your beliefs cements, or consummates, the relationship.

Immediately you will feel like the weight of the world has been lifted from you, and it has. Jesus does that—He loves you eternally and internally. Your next step is to seek and find an alive, Bible-based church. Ask around. I encourage you to read your Bible daily. Start in the Book of Proverbs then move on to the four Gospels. My two favorite Psalms are 34 and 112.

Be blessed! I will see you in Heaven,

—Dr. Bob

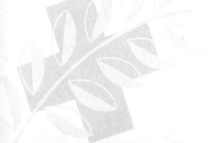

My Three-Month Goals

Take a moment, chew on what you have been doing the last twelve months, and project where you would like your life to be three months from now. Set physical, spiritual, emotional, and personal goals or targets.

_____

_____

_____

_____

_____

_____

_____

_____

_____

_____

_____

_____

_____

_____

_____

_____

_____

_____

My Six-Month Goals

Now that you have set and achieved a step in a new direction of *optimal health* what do you plan to do next?

_____

_____

_____

_____

_____

_____

_____

_____

_____

_____

_____

_____

_____

_____

_____

_____

_____

_____

My Twelve-Month Goals

In twelve months you will be the same person you are now, except to the degree that you act on what you have learned, books you have read, and people you have met. What is going to happen to you next? Think BIG—your new health level has set the foundation.

_____

_____

_____

_____

_____

_____

_____

_____

_____

_____

_____

_____

_____

_____

_____

_____

_____

My Five-Year Goals

Now that you have set short-term targets, what do you want to be part of your life in the next five years that will enhance and strengthen your optimal health lifestyle? Maybe enroll in health, nutrition or exercise classes; read more; share with others your optimal health knowledge? Jesus crossed over the sea to set free the man possessed with the demons. He acted; what are you going to be doing in five years?

_____

_____

_____

_____

_____

_____

_____

_____

_____

_____

_____

_____

_____

_____

_____

_____

_____

My Ten-Year Goals

Life speeds by. What you do now creates the foundation for future planning. Jesus created the mindset in His disciples to go to *all* the world. Are you ready to take the Gospel to your world? What will you be doing ten years from now?

_____

_____

_____

_____

_____

_____

_____

_____

_____

_____

_____

_____

_____

_____

_____

_____

_____

Endnotes

1. Janet Raloff, "Home Cooking on the Wane," *Science News* 162, no. 23 (December 2002): 7.

2. *New England Journal of Medicine* 346, no. 77 (2002): 124.

3. *American Medical Association* 292 (2004): 927.

4. *Annals Rheumatic Diseases* 59 (2000): 631.

5. Harvard School of Public Health, "Food Pyramids—What Should You Really Eat"? available from http://www.hsph.harvard.edu/nutritionsource/pyramids. html#references. See also *American Journal of Clinical Nutrition* 76 (2002): 1261-71.

6. *American Journal of Clinical Nutrition* 76 (2002): 1261.

7. *British Medical Journal* 325 (2002): 11.

8. *Strong's Expanded Dictionary of Bible Words* (Nelson Reference, 2001), #1657.

9. *International Journal of Obesity*, advance on-line publication (5 October 2004).

10. *Journal of the American Medical Association* 287 (2002): 356.

11. *New England Journal of Medicine* 345 (2001): 790.

12. *Ibid.*, 346 (2002): 393.

13. *Archives of Internal Medicine* 161 (2001): 2573.

14. *Journal of the American Dietary Association* 104 (2004): 1570.

15. *American Journal of Clinical Nutrition* 71 (2000): 921.

16. *Journal of the American Medical Association* 292 (2004): 1433.

17. *Ibid.,* 292 (2004): 1440.

18. *American Journal of Clinical Nutrition* 76 (2002): 1207.

19. Carol A. Nostrand, *Junk Food to Real Food, A Blueprint for Healthier Eating,* (Keats Publishing, 1994).

20. *Journal of the American Medical Association* 288 (2002): 3130.

21. *New England Journal of Medicine* 348 (2003): 2599, 2595.

22. *Strong's,* #5331.

23. *Obesity Research* 12 (2004): A23.

24. *New England Journal of Medicine* 351 (2004): 2694.

25. *American Journal of Clinical Nutrition* 81 (2005): 16.

26. *Journal of the American Medical Association* 293 (2005): 455.

27. *Diabetes Care* 27 (2004): 2993.

28. *Journal of the American Medical Association* 293 (2005): 86.

29. *American Journal of Clinical Nutrition* 80 (2004): 1492.

30. *American Medical Association* 287 (2002): 598.

31. *Journal of the American Medical Association* 295 (2006): 1539.

32. Susan Coburn, "Healthful topics: Treating Chronic Pain," Special to the *Stamford Advocate,* appeared in the *Chronicle Telegram* (Elyria, OH: June 1, 2003).

33. Bonnie Liebman, *New England Journal of Medicine* 343 (2000): 530, 572.

34. Susan M. Lark, "Fibrocystic Breast Disease," excerpt from *The Women's Health Companion* (Celestial Arts, Nutrition Action Newsletter).

35. *Journal of the American Medical Association* 288 (2002): 2554.

36. *American Journal Epidemiology* 159 (2004): 454.

37. *U.S. News & World Report* (January 23, 2001): 54.

38. Anthony Morrocco, "The 10 Most Unwanted List," *Grain and Salt News*, www
.celtic-seasalt.com.

39. *Journal of the National Cancer Institute* 95 (2003): 1079.

40. *Science* 307 (2005): 530, 584.

41. *Prostaglandins Leukot. Essent. Fatty Acids* 71 (2004): 153.

42. *Journal of the American Medical Association* 292 (2004): 1440.

43. *Ibid.*

44. *American Journal of Clinical Nutrition* 80 (2004): 38, 76.

45. *BL Archives of Pediatric and Adolescent Medicine* 154 (2000): 542, 610.

46. "Q: Do you want fries with that? A: Nope" *USA Today* (September 22, 2003),
and "A portion is a portion is a…." *The Plain Dealer* (January 29, 2003).

47. *Ins. J. Obes. Relat. Metab. Disord.* 28 (2004): 282.

48. *New England Journal of Medicine* 348 (2003): 977.

49. *Archives of Internal Medicine* 158 (1998): 2349.

50. *Journal of American Medical Association* 280 (1998): 1843.

51. *New England Journal of Medicine* 339 (1998): 785.

52. *Environmental Health Perspectives* 106, suppl. 3 (1998): 887.

53. *Journal of the American Medical Association* 269 (2003): 1785.

54. *New England Journal of Medicine* 350 (2004): 2542-2549.

55. *Nutrition Action Healthletter* (September 1999).

56. *Journal of Geriatric Psychiatry and Neurology* 9 (1996): 83.

57. *Physiology & Behavior* 62 (1997): 709.

58. *American Heart Journal* 150 (2005): 94.

59. Bonnie Liebman, *J. Amer. Med. Assoc.* 283 (2000): 2674.

60. *Hypertension* 38 (2001): 317.

61. *New England Journal of Medicine* 346 (2002): 393.

62. *American Medical Association* 292 (2004): 1447, 1454.

63. Bonnie Liebman, *New England Journal of Medicine* 341 (1999): 777, 836.

About Dr. Bob

Dr. Bob DeMaria is an experienced natural healthcare provider. He has focused his career on helping patients with drugless therapeutic protocols. Dr. Bob has a degree in human Biology, specialties in Spinal Engineering and Natural Orthopedic Treatment. He graduated cum laude and the valedictorian of his class. He practices clinically as a Chiropractor (DC). Dr. Bob continually pursues advanced educational opportunities and is currently studying to earn a Natural Health Doctor (NHD) degree.

Dr. Bob co-hosts a TV program with Deb, his wife of over thirty-five years. He has been a college instructor, team physician, business health consultant, and post-graduate trainer in the legal and health fields. He has written six other books, which are available at www.druglessdoctor.com. Dr. Bob also has several workshop audio series, "Dr. Bob's Top 10 Tips for Wellness."

Dr. Bob is an international speaker, has served as an expert witness, and has been in an active practice since 1978. He gave his life to the Lord in 1987. He and his wife appreciate the prayers of all who read this *Guide to Optimal Health*. He has two sons, Dominic and Anthony. A portion of the proceeds from this book will be used to financially support Bethany Blessing Ministry.

Dr. DeMaria is available on a limited basis to speak at your next Corporate Event or Convention. His energetic speaking style will inspire, educate and motivate your employees or downline to greater levels of health, wealth, and personal confidence. Dr. Bob's enthusiasm for life is **contagious!**

> Contact information:
>
> Phone: 1-888-922-5672
>
> Fax: 440-323-1566
>
> E-Mail: drbobdemaria@gmail.com

Bethany Blessing Ministry & Resources

Missionary Testimonies

Dennis and Mary Skinner: Three years ago we became full-time missionaries in the nation of Haiti. From the moment Dr. Bob and Debbie learned that we were leaving to minister in another country, they began to prayerfully and financially support us monthly, encouraged us through e-mail letters, and even saw to it that we received good, helpful Christian-living reading materials. Many times my wife and I were faced with difficult challenges and received sound counsel, wisdom, and Godly instruction from Dr. Bob and Debbie. The spiritual growth we have witnessed in both Dr. Bob and Debbie is attributed, in our opinion, to their relentless pursuit of God's purpose for their lives. Not only are they themselves charging toward the next level in Christ, but they are assisting others in that direction as well!

The Gordon family: Dr. Bob and Debbie have faithfully supported our family for several years. We minister in India. We have been able to touch many lives. Thanks to their support we have been relieved of additional time used to seek finances while serving our God-given purpose. Thank you for funding Bethany Blessing Ministry.

Rocky and Joske Malloy: We are active missionaries in Bolivia. The DeMaria family has graciously supported our endeavors, which at times has been near death. We have been blessed to penetrate the school system with Christian books. We continue to see the hand of God move in our lives. You will reap eternal blessings by supporting Bethany Blessing Ministry.

Partner With Us—Bethany Blessing Ministry

Bethany Blessing Ministry is a nonprofit organization based on Luke 24:50, "*And he* [Jesus] *led them out as far as to Bethany, and He lifted up his hands and blessed them.*" The ministry has several functions. One of the primary purposes is to establish locations for missionaries to rest while on leave from active duty in the field. We will provide a peaceful haven so the participants do not need to share a home or live in a hotel environment. There are those of you who have been called to be in active contact while others support the Kingdom of God with finances. For more information, visit www.BethanyBlessing.org.

Be a blessing. Be a part of the expansion of the Gospel to the whole world. Monthly partners will receive regular correspondence from the ministry. Please consider a monthly gift of $24 or $50 that will be used to further God's glory worldwide. All gifts are tax deductible.

You may copy the following page, complete the information, and Fax your donation to: 440-323-1566.

Or complete the page and mail it along with your check to:

Bethany Blessing Ministry

362 East Bridge Street

Elyria, OHIO 44035

Name: _____

Address: _____

City: _____ State: _____ Zip: _____

Telephone: _____

E-mail Address: _____

Payment: Check   Credit Card: Visa   MasterCard

Card number: _____

Exp. Date: _____

Name as Printed on Card: _____

Security Code: _____ Date: _____

Authorized Signature: _____

Dr. Bob Resources

I have been blessed to use a variety of products and surveys to improve the state of health for my patients. These items are available to you including the Hair Analysis, Saliva Testing, Symptom Survey, and Diet Journal Review. I also have a variety of natural nutritional supplements and products for you to choose from.

Supplementation (Available on-line at www.DruglessDoctor.com)

Bile: Produced in the liver. Needed for fat metabolism. Gallbladder removal necessitates a staircase approach to regular bile salt consumption. I encourage continued use.

B vitamins: Needed for nerve and fat function. Depleted by sugar consumption and stress. Symptoms include crying without reason.

B6 vitamin: Used by the body as a part of normal fat metabolism and brain function. Commonly deficient in sugar consumptions and birth control use. A deficiency is seen in low liver enzyme tests.

Zinc test: The zinc taste test is an interesting way to evaluate your zinc levels. I have found from my experience that low zinc is a body signal of various conditions that may need assistance. A good way to start your health program.

Other items are available to assist you in your health pursuit of *natural optimal health*. Visit www.DruglessDoctor.com and have a look around.

I also offer weekly online natural health workshops that I provide for my patients. You may purchase them to increase your knowledge; and they can be used as Continuing Education Credits (CEU) credits for many professions. Visit www.DruglessDoctor.com andand click on Health Guide/Journal.

Additional Services

Dr. Bob, or an associate, is available for personal consultation. Visit our Website at www.DruglessDoctor.com. These are not diagnostic consultations and are not meant to replace your personal healthcare provider.

E-Tips

Register at www.druglessdoctor.com

Follow us on Twitter @druglessdoctor

Facebook Dr. Bob: The Drugless Doctor

YouTube.com/druglessdoctor

Resources

Biotics Research Foundation

http://www.bioticsresearch.com

Biotics Research Corporation is a privately owned family business that adheres to the strictest quality control standards. I know from experience any of the oil products you select from them on our web site at www.druglessdoctor.com will make an impact on your overall health. I personally use their Bio Omega 3 anchovy and sardine formulated marine oil to supplement my oil intake and I use the Omega Nutrition Flax oil on my salads.

Omega Nutrition

www.omeganutrition.com

Omega Nutrition was developed after seeing the results of diets lacking in omega-3 fats. They are a company located both in Washington State and also in Canada. Omega Nutrition uses their patented Omegaflo system to cold press flax seeds and create a fresh, kosher GMO-free flax seed oil.

The Grain and Salt Company

www.celticseasalt.com

The Grain and Salt Society is a diverse company providing much more than only sea salt. Their large range of products includes Celtic Sea Salt, of course, teas, nut butters, and beauty products, just to name a few. Their salt is farmed in France, considered the richest supply in the world. Sea Salt is a favorite among chefs and The Grain and Salt Society's Celtic sea salt is Kosher, inspected by a rabbi who comes unannounced to ensure quality. Selina has been pursuing worldwide sources of quality new products. I thoroughly enjoy and use all of the seasonings.

Jordan Rubins

Author of *The Maker's Diet* and *Patient Heal Thyself*. Jordan overcame a debilitating illness and chronicles his journey *in Patient Heal Thyself*. His healthy eating choices are outlined in *The Maker's Diet*. Jordan is the founder of Garden of Life, provider of whole food supplements.

GAIA Herbs

www.gaiaherbs.com

GAIA Herbs is a North American Herb company that is defined by Purity + Integrity = Potency. How they proceed is as important as the produce. Each herb must be cultivated in accordance to nature's intent. As they create herbal medicines, they ensure the fullest possible expression of each herb. It is only through their dedication to purity and integrity that they deliver the powerful effects of each herb. I have used their herbs singly and as a proprietary blend helping our patients advance their over body function, reduce pain, and improve fat metabolism.

The Well Being Journal

www.wellbeingjournal.com

"We don't think we've seen the end of health."

The Well Being Journal is dedicated to publishing research about well-being and the integrity of medicine, which includes physical, mental, emotional, social and spiritual aspects of health and healing. The Journal has published, since 1992, research findings that substantiate the role in health of healthy thinking, good nutrition and nutritional supplements, traditional medicines, such as herbal, and the power of intent to heal, also called energy medicine and spiritual healing. Housed in our article archives are many personal stories of hope written by individuals who have healed from cancer, heart disease, arthritis and more by using a variety of natural healing methods.

BOOKS BY DR. BOB

DR. BOB'S DRUGLESS GUIDE TO DETOXIFICATION

This may be the most toxic time in history. Daily headlines report the negative conditions of our water, food, and air. The "green movement" is popularly creating a mindset to secure a safer, cleaner environment, but little is said about the circumstances our bodies have to contend with. This book is a logical plan that establishes true wellness in your body from the inside out. Dr. Bob shares clinically proven, time-tested protocols that can be followed in the comfort of your own home—no need to travel to expensive clinics or follow strict and stressful diet plans.

You will learn what to purchase at your own grocery store to maintain a healthy body, be empowered to make wise choices and not be dependent on medications, avert possible surgical intervention to remove an exhausted dysfunctional organ, and learn what to eat and what to avoid to create an optimally functioning cellular environment!

DR. BOB'S GUIDE TO STOP ADHD IN 18 DAYS
A Drugless Family Guide to Optimal Health

Anyone can successfully overcome ADHD and Hyperactivity without drugs. This book details how to get your children and family off medications and detrimental junk foods filled with trans fatty acids, dairy products, sugar and preservatives, so that they can have optimal, natural health. This is a simple, effective step-by-step plan that includes adding FLAX OIL and modifying your diet and vitamin/mineral intake. The protocol will improve your nervous system function, and help you overcome behavioral and learning problems. It will improve insomnia, mood swings and irritability. The result will be your body healing itself naturally. Participants in the pilot program saw improvement in only 18 days. NATURALLY!

DR. BOB'S DRUGLESS GUIDE TO BALANCING FEMALE HORMONES

The time tested information in this book is designed to create a state of optimal health in the female hormonal system. Dr. Bob's insight into cell function will empower the reader to make wise choices designed to nourish and detoxify the body with items that can be easily incorporated in a day-to-day routine. You will learn that a clear and clean lymphatic system is important and that a functioning liver is vital for balance. The role of nutrients like iodine and proper oil help create the foundation needed to progress into hormonal maturity without annoying body signals. You will be exposed to the procedures that Dr. Bob has used to transition his patients into feeling great without medication.

DR. BOB & DEBBIE'S GUIDE TO SEX AND ROMANCE

Dr. Bob and Debbie's Guide to Sex and Romance is a collection of personal and clinically based evidence including protocols applied and successfully used from Dr. Bob's health care practice. Dr. Bob and Debbie also share their commonsense experience from 40 years of their personal relationship and over 30 years of marriage. You will gain from the insight they have gleaned from their involvement and observations discovered while being in Natural Health since 1978. The DeMarias have watched the decline of the overall personal health of the new patients presented to the clinic and discuss the restoration of those individuals' overall health. Dr. Bob linked the associated deterioration of sexual desire and whole body dysfunction with patients having chronic health challenges.

DR. BOB'S MEN'S HEALTH—THE BASICS

Dr. Bob's Men's Health—The Basics is for men who want simple, honest answers to their basic health questions. In today's culture women tend to make the majority of the healthcare decisions for their families—while men tend to avoid seeking care, often times, until the pain and discomfort caused by the conditions they have suffered with are beyond their ability to cope with. Dr. Bob's extensive experience as a healthcare provider, without the use of prescription medication, has provided him with a unique ability to understand and relay logical solutions in an easy to follow format. In this book, Dr. Bob reveals important, little known facts on the more common conditions men contend with: heart disease, cancer, cholesterol, sexual dysfunction and pain. You will learn the basics which will propel you to levels of optimal health, without the use of prescription medication.

DR. BOB'S TRANS FAT SURVIVAL GUIDE
Why No Fat, Low Fat, Trans Fat is KILLING YOU!

This book explains the dangers of trans fat, commonly called hydrogenated and partially hydrogenated fat, as well as how to recognize it in everyday food by properly reading nutritional labels. Along with trans fat, you will learn the different types of fats, which ones are beneficial, and which ones should be used for cooking, baking, or eating. Not to leave the reader hanging with questions on how to eliminate dangerous fats and take on a healthier approach to life, there are several sections dealing with how to make those changes, transitioning healthier foods into their eating plan. This book will encourage and empower you to make better choices and learn to live an optimal and healthy life.